PREMENOPAUSE & MENOPAUSE

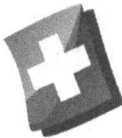

HealthScouter

WWW.HEALTHSCOUTER.COM

HealthScouter.com - Equity Press
5055 Canyon Crest Drive
Riverside, California 92507
www.healthscouter.com

Purchasing this book entitles you to free updates at
www.healthscouter.com/menopause

Edited By: Mark P. Schmitz

Includes Menopause from Wikipedia
http://en.wikipedia.org/wiki/Menopause

Menopause and Premenopause: A Menopause Patient Self Advocacy Guide: HealthScouter Menopause: Menopause Symptoms and Menopause Treatment

ISBN 978-1-60332-067-2

Important

NEVER DISREGARD PROFESSIONAL MEDICAL ADVICE, OR DELAY SEEKING IT, BECAUSE OF SOMETHING YOU HAVE READ IN THIS BOOK. ALWAYS SEEK PROFESSIONAL MEDICAL ADVICE BEFORE ACTING UPON INFORMATION READ IN THIS BOOK.

HealthScouter and Equity Press do not provide medical advice. The contents of this book are for informational purposes only and are not intended to substitute for professional medical advice, diagnosis or treatment. Always seek advice from a qualified physician or health care professional about any medical concern, and do not disregard professional medical advice because of anything you may read in this book or on a HealthScouter Web site. The views of individuals quoted in this book are not necessarily those of HealthScouter or Equity Press.

While this book is intended to be a medium for the exchange of information and ideas, it is not meant in any way to be a substitute for sound medical advice; neither should it be viewed as a trusted source of such advice. The views expressed in these messages are not those of any qualified medical association, and the publisher is not responsible for the validity of the information communicated herein or for consequences that may arise from acting upon this information. The publisher is not responsible for any content found in the book that may be deemed offensive, inappropriate, inaccurate or medically unsound. The information you find here is only for the purpose of discussion and should not be the basis for any medical decision. The content is not intended to be a substitute for professional medical advice, diagnosis or treatment.

The information presented is not to be considered complete, nor does it contain all medical resource information that may be relevant, and therefore it is not intended to be a substitute for seeking medical treatment and/or appropriate care.

By reading this book and parts of the Web site, you agree under all circumstances to hold harmless, and to refrain from seeking remedy from, the owners of this book. The publisher shall disclaim all liability to you for damages, costs or expenses, including legal and medical fees, related to your reliance on anything derived from this book or Web site or its contents. Furthermore, Equity Press assumes no liability for any and all claims arising out of the said use, regardless of the cause, effects, or fault.

Equity Press and HealthScouter do not endorse any company or product, and listing on the HealthScouter Web site is not linked to corporate sponsorship. We do not make a claim to being comprehensive or up to date. If you would like to recommend information to include in this book, please contact us – we would be very happy to hear from you.

Purchasing this book entitles you to free updates as they are available. Please register your book at www.healthscouter.com/menopause

Table of Contents

Menopause

Menopause

From Wikipedia, the free encyclopedia

Menopause is the permanent shutting down of the female reproductive system in mammals, including humans.

The word was first applied to humans, and because of this it literally means the cessation of monthly cycles or menstrual cycles, from the Greek roots *meno* (month) and *pausis* (cessation). However, the word is not only applied to humans, and menopause is the permanent stopping of female reproductive cycles of various lengths and kinds; menopause is indeed present in a number of mammal species other than humans.

In adult human females who still have a uterus, and who are not pregnant or lactating, postmenopause is identified by a permanent (at least one year's) absence of monthly periods or menstruation. In women without a uterus, menopause or postmenopause is identified by a very high FSH level.

In human females, menopause usually happens more or less in midlife, signaling the end of the fertile phase of a woman's life. Menopause is perhaps most easily understood as the opposite process to menarche, the start of the monthly periods. However, menopause in women cannot satisfactorily be defined simply as the permanent "stopping of the monthly periods", because in reality what is happening to the uterus is quite secondary to the process; it is what is happening to the ovaries that is the crucial factor.

For medical reasons, the uterus must sometimes be surgically removed (hysterectomy) in a younger woman; her periods will cease permanently, and the woman will technically be infertile, but as long as at least one of her ovaries is still functioning, the woman will *not* have entered menopause; even without the uterus, ovulation and the release of the sequence of reproductive hormones will continue to cycle on until menopause is reached. But in circumstances when a woman's ovaries are removed (oophorectomy), even if the uterus were to be left intact, the woman will immediately be in "surgical menopause".

Thus menopause is based on the natural or surgical cessation of hormone production by the ovaries, which are a part of the body's endocrine system of hormone production, in this case the hormones which make reproduction possible and may influence sexual behavior. The resultant decreased levels of circulating estrogen impacts entire cascade of a woman's reproductive functioning, from brain to skin.

The menopause transition, and postmenopause itself, is a natural life change, not a disease state or a disorder. The transition itself can be challenging for a number of women, but for others it is not difficult.

Overview

Menopause starts as the ovaries begin to alter in their function and the egg, surrounded by its follicles (which, during the menstrual years, leads to ovulation and menstruation if pregnancy does not occur), slows and becomes unpredictable. This may lead to skipped periods (eventually) and other perimenopausal symptoms, gradually leading to the end of the fertile phase of a woman's life. After a number of years of erratic functioning, the ovaries almost completely stop producing progesterone and two out of the three estrogen hormones: estradiol and estriol. Estrone is one estrogen which is still produced in reasonable amounts in post-menopausal women. Testosterone levels decrease; however, a decrease in testosterone levels begins gradually in young adulthood. Testosterone levels are thought not to drop significantly during the menopause transition because the stroma of the post-menopausal ovary and the adrenal gland still continue to secrete small amounts of testosterone, even during postmenopause.

Menopause is the end of the reproductive years rather than the beginning, and thus it is the opposite of menarche, nonetheless it can usefully be compared with that event: the menopause transition years are in many ways similar to puberty in reverse, and the psychological and social challenges of the Change are also somewhat similar to those encountered during adolescence.

Age of onset

The average age of menopause in the Western world is 51 years, and the normal age range for the occurrence of menopause is somewhere between the age of 45 and 55. The last period ever occurring between the ages of 55 to 60 is known as a "late menopause." An "early menopause" on the other hand is defined as the last period ever between the age of 40 to 45.

Rarely the ovaries stop working at a very early age, anywhere from the age of puberty to age 40, and this is known as premature ovarian failure (POF), also commonly referred to as "premature menopause." One percent of women experience POF, and it is not considered to be due to the normal effects of aging.

Some known causes of premature menopause include autoimmune disorders, thyroid disease, diabetes mellitus, chemotherapy, and radiotherapy. However, in the majority of spontaneous cases of premature menopause, the cause is unknown.

Premature menopause is diagnosed or confirmed by measuring the levels of follicle-stimulating hormone (FSH) and luteinizing hormone (LH); the levels of these hormones will be abnormally high if menopause has occurred. Rates of premature menopause have been found to be significantly higher in fraternal and identical twins; approximately 5 percent of twins reach menopause before the age of 40. The reasons for this are not completely understood. Transplants of ovarian tissue between identical twins have been successful in restoring fertility.

Menopause in other species

Menopause in the animal kingdom appears perhaps to be somewhat uncommon, although the incidence in different species has by no means been thoroughly researched. However, it is already quite apparent that humans are not the only species that experience it. Menopause has been observed in rhesus monkeys[1], some cetaceans[2], as well as in a variety of other species of vertebrates including the guppy, the platyfish, the budgerigar, the laboratory rat and mouse, the opossum, and all manner of primates[3].

Menopause in human evolution

The Grandmother hypothesis suggests that menopause evolved in humans because it promotes the survival of grandchildren. According to this hypothesis, post-reproductive women feed and care for children, adult nursing daughters, and grandchildren whose mothers have weaned them. Human babies require large and steady supplies of glucose to feed the growing brain. In infants in the first year of life, the brain consumes 60 percent of all calories, so both babies and their mothers require a dependable food supply. Some evidence suggests that hunters contribute less than half the total food budget of most hunter-gatherer societies, and often much less than half, so that foraging grandmothers can contribute substantially to the survival of grandchildren at times when mothers and fathers are unable to gather enough food for all the children. In general, selection operates most powerfully during times of famine or other privation. So although grandmothers might not be necessary during good times, many grandchildren cannot survive without them during times of famine.

Social and psychological significance

The shutting down of the female reproductive system in midlife ushers in the third part of a woman's life. Many women in Western culture live long enough that half of their adult life is spent in postmenopause. The menopause transition is a major life change, similar to menarche in the magnitude of its social and psychological significance. In the ancient past, menarche and menopause were considered to mark the transitions from "maiden" to "matron", and from "matron" to "crone". Whereas the significance of the changes that surround menarche is still fairly well recognized, in countries such as the USA, the social and psychological ramifications of the menopause transition are frequently ignored or underestimated.

Terminology, definitions and commentary

Menopause

Clinically speaking, menopause is a date: for those women who still have a uterus, menopause is defined as the day after a woman's final period finishes. This date is fixed retrospectively, once 12 months have gone by with no menstrual flow at all.

In common everyday parlance however, the word "menopause" is usually not used to refer to one day, but to the whole of the menopause transition years. This span of time is also referred to as the **change of life**, the **change**, or the **climacteric** and more recently is known as "perimenopause" (literally meaning "around menopause").

Perimenopause

In biomedicine, perimenopause means the menopause transition years. In women who have a uterus, perimenopause is the years both before and after the final period (although it is only possible to determine retroactively which episode of flow was indeed the final period). During perimenopause, the production of most of the reproductive hormones, including the estrogens, progesterone and testosterone, diminishes and becomes more irregular, often with wide and unpredictable fluctuations in levels. During this period, fertility diminishes, but is not considered to reach zero until the official date of menopause is reached, and this date, as previously mentioned, can only be determined retrospectively. Signs and effects of the menopause transition can begin as early as age 35, although most women who become aware of the transition do so about ten years later, often in their mid to late 40s. The duration of perimenopause with noticeable bodily effects can be a few years, ten years or even longer. The actual duration and severity of perimenopause in any individual woman cannot be predicted in advance or during the process.

In the perimenopause years, many women find that they undergo some bodily effects resulting from hormonal fluctuation, such as hot flashes. When these effects are strong, women may sometimes seek medical advice. Mood changes, insomnia, fatigue, memory problems, and other complaints are sometimes considered to be unrelated to the hormonal fluctuations, but not enough research has been done to properly clarify any of these issues. However, for cultural reasons, even women who are free of any troublesome physical effects of perimenopause, may nonetheless find themselves moving through a psychosocial transition.

One piece of recent research appears to show that melatonin supplementation in perimenopausal women can produce a highly significant improvement in thyroid function and gonadotropin levels, as well as restoring fertility and menstruation and preventing the depression associated with the menopause[4].

Perimenopause is a relatively new term. The use of it was criticized by some cultural commentators, because they feel that it extends the negative connotations of menopause (namely symptomology) over many more years of a woman's life.

Premenopause

Premenopause is a word used to describe the years leading up to the last period ever, when the levels of reproductive hormones are already becoming lower and more erratic, and the effects of hormone withdrawal may be present.

Postmenopause

Postmenopause is all of the time in a woman's life that take place after her last period ever, or more accurately, all of the time that follows the point when her ovaries become inactive. A woman who still has her uterus can be declared to be in postmenopause once she has gone 12 full months with no flow at all, not even any spotting. When she reaches that point, she is one year into postmenopause. The reason for this delay in declaring a woman postmenopausal is because periods are usually extremely erratic at this time of life, and therefore a reasonably long stretch of time is necessary to be sure that the cycling has actually ceased completely. In women who have no uterus, and therefore have no periods, postmenopause can be determined by a blood test which can reveal the very high levels of follicle-stimulating hormone (FSH) that are typical of post-menopausal women. A woman's reproductive hormone levels continue to drop and fluctuate for some time into postmenopause, so any hormone withdrawal symptoms that a woman may be experiencing do not necessarily stop right away, but may take quite some time, even several years, to disappear completely. Any period-like flow that might occur during postmenopause, even just spotting, must be reported to a doctor. The cause may in fact be minor, but the possibility of endometrial cancer must be checked for and eliminated.

The causes of Menopause

The causes of menopause can be considered from complementary proximate (mechanistic) and ultimate (adaptive evolutionary) perspectives.

From a proximate perspective

A natural or physiological menopause is that which occurs as a part of a woman's normal aging process. It is the result of the eventual atresia of almost all oocytes in the ovaries. This causes an increase in circulating follicle-stimulating hormone (FSH) and luteinizing hormone (LH) levels as there are a decreased number of oocytes responding to these hormones and producing estrogen. This decrease in the production of estrogen leads to the perimenopausal symptoms of hot flashes, insomnia and mood changes, as well as post-menopausal osteoporosis and vaginal atrophy.

However, menopause can be surgically induced by bilateral salpingo-oophorectomy (removal of both ovaries and both fallopian tubes), which is often, but not always, done in conjunction with hysterectomy. Cessation of menses as a result of removal of the ovaries is called "surgical menopause". The sudden and complete drop in reproductive hormone levels usually produces extreme hormone-withdrawal symptoms such as hot flashes, etc.

As mentioned above, removal of the uterus, hysterectomy, does not itself cause menopause, although pelvic surgery can sometimes precipitate a somewhat earlier menopause, perhaps because of a compromised blood supply to the ovaries. Removing the ovaries, however, causes an immediate and powerful "surgical menopause", even if the uterus is left intact.

Cigarette smoking has been found to decrease the age at menopause by as much as one year, and women who have undergone hysterectomy with ovary conservation go through menopause 3.7 years earlier than average. However, premature menopause (before the age of 40) is generally idiopathic.

From an ultimate perspective

(An ultimate perspective on menopause is above in the "Menopause in human evolution" section.)

Possible effects of perimenopause, the menopause transition time

As the body responds to the rapidly changing levels of natural hormones, a number of effects can appear. It is however worth pointing out, that not every woman experiences bothersome levels of these effects, and even in those women who do experience strong effects, the range of effects and the degree to which they appear is very variable from person to person. Those effects that are due to low estrogen levels (for example vaginal atrophy and skin drying) remain present even after the menopause transition years are over; however, many of the effects that are caused by the extreme fluctuations in hormone levels (for example hot flashes and mood changes) usually disappear or improve significantly once the perimenopause transition time has been completed.

Both users and non-users of hormone replacement therapy identify lack of energy as the most frequent and distressing effect[5] Other effects can include vasomotor symptoms such as hot flashes and palpitations, psychological effects such as depression, anxiety, irritability, mood swings, memory problems and lack of concentration, and atrophic effects such as vaginal dryness and urgency of urination.

The average woman also has increasingly erratic menstrual periods, due to skipped ovulations. Typically the timing of the flow becomes unpredictable. In addition the duration of the flow may be considerably shorter or longer than normal, and the flow itself may be significantly heavier or lighter than was previously the case, including sometimes long episodes of spotting. Early in the process it is not uncommon to have some two-week cycles. Further into the process it is common to skip periods for months at a time, and these skipped periods may be followed by a heavier period. The number of skipped periods in a row often increases as the time of last period approaches. As mentioned above, when a woman of menopausal age has not had a period or any spotting for 12 months, at that point she is considered to be one year into postmenopause. However, a period after six months of no flow at all is sometimes considered worthy of investigation by a doctor.

All the various possible perimenopause effects are caused by an overall drop, as well as dramatic but erratic fluctuations, in the absolute levels and relative levels of estrogens and progesterone. Some of the effects, such as formication, may be associated directly with hormone withdrawal.

Vasomotor instability

- hot flashes or hot flushes, including night sweats and, in a few people, cold flashes

I thought I was going nuts. I was having hot flashes, and then here come these cold periods where I'm wearing a robe in June. Sometimes it feels like I have a low-grade fever. Then at night I have the hot flashes.

I have suffered with this low-grade fever feeling, and it really made me very anxious as to what was going on. My doctor used to look at me as if I were a mad hypochondriac, so it is nice in a strange way to know others who have had this also have fibromyalgia, IBS, and acid reflux. These have been with me for about five years. I am now able to blame the menopause. I suffer hot and sweaty bouts and have just had blood work done to see if my thyroid is abnormal, as my symptoms tend to last for ages and are very regular.

I feel hot inside but my skin is cold. I have this when I'm on my periods. It's like I have a constant fever and hot feet when in bed. I also wake up soaking wet, with sweat, when periods end it stops. I'm 48, it worries me that I have a fever and there's something wrong with me. I thought a flash was a flash but this stays for hours. Because of persistent nausea, I had a full battery of tests a few years ago, including an Endoscopic Ultrasound, which showed nothing. After finding these boards (and having all tests come back negative), I am sure this is all perimenopause-related.

When I first started menopause, I had severe hot flashes and sweated buckets. I thought I was going to go insane when a hot flash hit me. And at the moment it started, I had this intense feeling to drink anything I could get my hands on. When you get thirsty, that means you are already dehydrated and your body is telling you to drink. I always have a bottle of seltzer water on hand when the hot flashes start coming back to back. The warmer weather always brings them on more. I never drank so much water and seltzer since this madness started. But the good news is those severe flashes calm down a lot as your body adjusts to all the changes. Then you just have those annoying ones. Try to drink as often as you can to ward off dehydrating. Try not to worry over this. You will be okay. This is very normal. And to think I couldn't wait for my cycles to end. I would give anything to have them back again.

Last spring I started what I thought was menopause and went 180+ days without a period and miserable dripping wet hot flashes/night sweats. Then I started periods again every 19 days which lasted eight to ten days. Now I am again 100+ days into no periods and hot flashes/night sweats are back. Is this normal as one enters full menopause to have no cycles and then some and then not again? I am 46 years old and have been experiencing perimenopause symptoms (irregular periods and stuff) for about the past ten years. Does anyone else experience hot flashes with changes in environment (like going from outside to inside), etc., and does physical exertion make them worse? I've tried different herbal remedies and stuff to relieve the hot flashes, but with no success. I am not a candidate for HRT, because of my immediate family history (my mother, who had hormone related breast cancer) and do not want to risk taking HRT.

My periods have been completely erratic since the beginning of February. I had one period and then didn't have one for nearly 39 days. In March I had a very short period, stopped for four days, then came on again for three days and felt strange cramping in my abdomen. (During the whole cycle, I felt exhausted and sick.) Then I had two-and-a-half wonderful weeks on holiday in the sun and came back to complete exhaustion and another period. This only lasted three days and then I got more cramping as though another period wanted to come on but didn't! This is all completely crazy and erratic.

I've been having night sweats on and off for the last year or so (I'm 45). Lately I've had profuse night sweating in the genital area. I'll wake up in the middle of the night drenched in sweat from my belly button to mid-thigh. It's so bad that my bed gets all damp from it, so in the morning I have to pull everything off to air it (and yes, it definitely is sweat, not anything else). I still sweat in other areas, too, but that particular area is just SO bad. In this same time, I've had frequent yeast infections and milia, most likely because the area is just not as dry as it should be.

I am in perimenopause still and have a pretty regular cycle, so far. I get occasional hot flashes, but I don't really sweat. I get bright red. If you are looking at me, you can see it rise up my neck to my face. Sometimes the heat is so intense; it makes me a little nauseous. I know of one friend who didn't really have any of the symptoms, ever. She went through perimenopause and menopause in about five years and was done! I know that will not be my future. I just saw my gynecologist last week for my annual and he said it is so unpredictable from woman to woman. Even though the symptoms are the same, the time frames and the number and intensity of symptoms is usually an individual thing. I learned something interesting though. I started puberty really young. I was nine years old. So I figured I'd go through menopause early, too. My gynecologist said it's just the opposite. The earlier you start, the later you stop and vice versa.

I'm pretty sure I am perimenopausal. Among other symptoms, I've been having night sweats for the last couple of years on and off. I am getting these little pimples all over my chest and breasts. I think that it may be because of the sweating. That is the area where I seem to soak my shirt the worst every night. The problem is that the pimples that occur on my breasts leave scars. My hypothesis is that it is because the skin in that area is more sensitive and thinner than other places. I don't try to squeeze them, but they still scar. So now I have these little red dots all over my breasts, and this isn't attractive. My husband and I are the only ones to see them, but still...

I am going through perimenopause right now. I am 43 and I get hot flashes in the night and throw all my clothes off. I have always suffered from anxiety, and now with the hormone changes I have even had panic attacks in the night and gone to the emergency room. It's awful. My body feels like it is morphing into something strange. I have weird thoughts sometimes and fuzzy brain, like forgetful and stuff. I am even clumsy at times. I have weird twitches in my muscles right now that we can't figure out. My thyroid went out of whack, and I have been hypothyroid for two years. That has been a pain to get leveled out. I am the only one in my family with this disorder. My calcium level is low and I have had to get on supplements now. The whole thing is just freaking me out and I feel so alone. My husband doesn't understand. How can he? I bought some natural things to try, such as liquid vitamins that get right into your bloodstream. I also bought some progesterone cream, but I have only tried it for two days.

I have had the eye twitching before. My daughter works for eye doctors and they said it could be from changing hormones or too much caffeine. It isn't a serious problem, just really annoying. My chin started to twitch about a week ago and it's still going strong. My girlfriend changed from synthetic hormone replacement to bioidentical hormones a while back, and during that time she said every muscle in her face started twitching, which leads me to believe hormones must have a lot to do with it.

I have had internal trembling and shaking for a year now and some days it is very mild and other days it's worse. I also notice that when I am painting my nails, sometimes my fingers shake. Do you get that, too, or is it just internal only? I have the internal as well when my fingers kind of shake a little.

Well, I just started this trembling business in March, and I had been very worried about it until reading some of the entries on old threads. It's been comforting to know that others have this trembling/vibrating, too! My pharmacist mentioned that it could be related to menopause and hormones, so maybe it is. Mine started when I woke up at 3:00 a.m. vibrating from the waist up! Since then, it just stays with me. Sometimes others can see my hand tremble, but most of the time I just feel it inside. It's a very weird thing that I've never heard anyone relate to menopause before.

I have experienced an annoying "twitching feeling" mostly in my ankles/feet. It's usually when I'm sitting down after I walked a lot or when I lay down to go to sleep. I don't have this every day, but often enough that it bothers me. I am postmenopausal and was wondering if anyone else is having this problem. My doctor seems to know nothing (really!). I get B12 shots for a complicated deficiency, and the doctor says everything else is okay, even though he hasn't checked anything other than my B12 level every four months. I was thinking maybe I need iron, but he says I don't because my hemoglobin is good.

I have this "internal shaking", which at first felt like I had low blood sugar and I needed some food in me, but it has come and gone for the past five years (I am 51 and this all started when I was 47). It goes with the anxiety, which is the worst symptom for me. I had periods stop for a year, then had one, then stop for a year, and now just had one again. My hot flashes and stuff go away when I have my cycle start up, but the anxiety stays most of the time. Sometimes I wake up in the morning and I have this shaking hit me really hard. It's a drag. I really worried about it when it first started, but since I have found these boards I see it is another symptom of menopause for so many women and I have relaxed a bit about all the weird stuff.

I had the "trembling" or rather internal shaking sensations before and for a much longer time than the tingling left foot. The foot thing was one of the last things I had that was weird to me. The internal trembling was really scary and unbearable. It hit me hard, especially in the middle of the night when my whole body would be vibrating inside and would last for hours, even way into morning sometimes. I got to the point where I was scared to go to sleep each night, not knowing what I was to happen to me in the middle of the night. At that time, I didn't know of any women having this and my doctor was clueless. They really should include this symptom in more perimenopause symptoms lists and books.

The internal buzzing has been a big thing with me. It started back in August and was one of the first signs that I was starting the perimenopause, although at the time I had not developed any other symptoms and so wasn't aware what it was. It was really bad some days, and in the end I went to the doctor who referred me for a brain MRI. This came back normal, but the buzzing continued. It moves around my body, sometimes in my spine, sometimes pelvic region, legs, neck, etc. Finally I started to get other classic symptoms of perimenopause (fatigue, irregular periods, nausea, and feeling of warm in my face, etc.) and discovered this site. I hadn't realized what a common symptom it is during the perimenopause. Sometimes I am lying in bed and the vibrations are so strong it feels like an electric current is passing through my body. Other days I hardly get it at all. Magnesium seems to help and B vitamins.

For about the last ten days, I have felt pretty good again (after nearly 18 months of all the horrible menopause symptoms). I still get an odd hot flush and a bit of the internal shaking. But the depression, anxiety, strange feelings, foggy head, insomnia, sheer tiredness, lack of motivation and confidence, etc., have definitely lifted. Now I don't know if it's just coincidence, or maybe my body is just learning to adjust to the hormone imbalance, but I have been taking high strength evening primrose oil each day for about a fortnight, and I also started having a glass of soy milk every day after I had read that Chinese and Japanese women hardly get any menopause symptoms because their diets are so rich in soy.

My hot flashes seem to be more frequent and are lasting longer. When I am at work and it happens, I either go outside or find the nearest piece of paper to fan myself. For the last couple of months, mainly in the evenings, I am getting major cold flashes. If I get off the couch and go into the kitchen or something, I just freeze. It is miserable. This morning when I was in the shower, it was all I could do to wash my hair and body. The fatigue in the mornings is awful.

I guess my perimenopause started four years ago, when these awful palpitations started. I saw a cardiologist and had an ultrasound of my heart, numerous EKGs, chest x-ray, etc. All the results came back fine, and they said that I had an ectopic heartbeat. I have lived with it, but it has become worse again. At the same time as my periods are erratic, I have anxiety and numerous other problems. I would just like to describe my palpitations to see what you think: Sometimes I have the feeling of a missed beat or of an extra hard beat (the ectopic beat I was diagnosed with); a lot of the time it just feels like it is beating faster than normal—the most it gets up to is 85 bpm. The doctor says this is fine, but it feels horrible. Sometimes all these feelings happen together and then it is really weird. Should I trust that my heart is okay, seeing as the doctors said it was and it has managed another four years? Could it all be perimenopause as I suspect. I am 41 years old, but I feel 61!

Sometimes my heart is beating so fast my whole body pulsates with each beat. Sometimes it feels like it is beating up into my throat. Other times, I can hardly even feel it and then it is very slow but hard. When I get out of bed in the middle of the night, my heart will race and I sweat. I have had numerous work-ups over the years, as this started a long time ago. I even had one cardiologist ask me if I was using cocaine. My intern asked me if I had a pacemaker. I finally found a cardiologist who put me through the ultrasound of the heart and stress test. I had already worn the Holter monitor for 24 hours and used the device that is placed against the heart so when an episode occurs, it records it. For those not familiar with this, every time something happens, you record it and then dial a phone number and play the recording over the phone. If there is anything dangerous, an ambulance will be dispatched; otherwise, they keep track of what is going on for a month. The last couple of years, the palpitations were getting really bad when I went through menopause. I was already tweaked about my heart, as my dad died when he was 46 years old. Nothing I have is life-threatening. It is described as a little extra electrical impulse, like an extra beat. I take Digoxin now to help with the palpitations, but reassurance was a big deal to me. Avoiding caffeine helps, too. If you are having an episode, coughing sometimes helps and dipping your face in cold water, too. And I thought menopause meant simply no more periods.

I am 50 but I started noticing changes in my cycle around the age of 45 or 46 I think. I had palpitations around that time, too, if not a bit before. Everything checked out fine and they said my electrolytes were low and to drink more water, which I did and do now. I read that it is a symptom of perimenopause (palpitations), and so I think that is what that was all about. The intestinal stuff did not happen until these past couple years. But my stomach has always been sensitive and acting up around my period, and also my PMS has always been bad. My gynecologist said whatever I had in PMS before will be more pronounced during perimenopause, and I have found that to be so. I still have my period and do not see any big changes in that as far as it going a long time before I get one. A year ago or so it came on day 40 and then another time on day 50, but other than that it has been where it comes anywhere from day 23 to 34. (the last two times on day 34). I had detailed the symptoms I have had and still have and those I do not have as much of anymore. But suffice to say, some days are better than others in the perimenopause world for me!

I wish the hot flashes would disappear after a year. I remember my best friend would fan herself for a minute and indicate she was having a hot flash. Well, I wish that was all I experienced. It is like a bucket of water being thrown at me. My face and neck get red. My neck itches. I have sweat that runs down my face. It is just lovely. People looking at me have their eyes bulge when they see what I am going through. I can't hide it, so I just say I am having a little hot flash. I have to sleep on a towel at night because I sweat so much. I don't wear solid color shirts in case I start sweating. I have to admit the last month it hasn't been too bad, but I did go through an easier time about a year ago and then the sweats returned. I am in my third year. I won't take anything, as I have heard it only delays the symptoms. My mom had breast cancer, and I am not active enough to prevent blood clots, so I just grunt at how easy men have it and carry on.

I know I am about to have a flash when my stomach feels like its flipping over. I get nauseous, my nerve endings feel like they are standing on edge, I get a fight-or-flight feeling, and I get a squirmy feeling all over. Immediately after this, I get the hot flash. I have this same sequence of events every time, and sometimes I get a little light headed.

I have a warning right before a hot flash—my stomach does a little dance, I feel like I am having an anxiety issue, and then the hot flash comes on. It comes from the inside out and makes my head, neck, and back extremely hot and sweaty. My face and neck turn very red. It can last from one to three minutes, depending on what I have been doing. I have been on HRT for over two years, and HRT helped take these symptoms away. I am weaning off HRT, so I have many symptoms a day again along with night sweats. Everyone I have talked to that has been on and off a HRT has to go through all this anyway. So I am going to try and deal with it now and get it over.

I was thin when I started menopause and had hot flashes. Three years later, I am now 30 pounds overweight and still have hot flashes. I shouldn't call them flashes—they are more like a soaking. I am so sick of it. My newest "thing" is edema, and I think that is a lot of my weight gain. I just had blood work done today, but my new doctors aid it could be just from menopause. Egad, is everything caused by menopause?

Weight gain, unfortunately, is something we find happens, especially in your belly. From what I have learned about it, it's our metabolism when it, for some reason, decides to up and slow down, making it easier to gain and harder than all getout to lose. I found that I have gained a lot in my mid-section, making it hard to fit into my britches or at the very least look good in anything I wear. I have a round paunch that makes me look pregnant, and it's not a soft flab. It's sort of on the firmer side. And no, I am definitely not pregnant, just in case you were wondering. At nearly 50, I'd freak out if I were, but I had my tubes cut and tied 17 years ago.

I had a partial hysterectomy in 2000, they removed the uterus and one ovary. Early in 2006, I had the last ovary removed. I was put on Premarin 1.25 mg. for over a year. My mother died very suddenly from breast cancer last year, and I decided to get off the HRT because of the increased risk to me. It has been two-and-a-half months and my hot flashes and night sweats are so bad. I have used progesterin cream as well as black cohosh and nothing seems to help. I will have three to five an hour with extreme flushing. People are making comments about the color in my neck and face. It is so embarrassing as well as uncomfortable. I keep my house so cold that my husband and son are miserable. I am not sleeping at night because I have these flashes so often. I am beginning to wonder if it is worth the risk of cancer to have some quality of life at this time.

I have been on Premarin for ten years and my doctor decided I needed to either be off or tapered to a lower dose. So I tapered for months and finally I went off, and man you would of thought someone lit me on fire and forgot to turn it off! Holy cow I was hot so hot I thought I was going to explode, and this went on and on and on, month after month, and finally I said enough! The doctor looked for all kinds of reasons for my extreme heat, and I was tested for all kinds of strange stuff. Meanwhile my heat continue, so my doctor gave up and put me back on Premarin and I went back to being a human. Not doing that again! I still use a fan at night to keep the air circulating, which makes sleeping pleasant. In 10+ years I have not had any side effects from Premarin, so I really don't care how long I have to be on it. I just don't think I should have to go through torture just because medical science has all the doctors up a tree.

I have terrible hot flushes at the moment, unbearable at times, but like the others I make a joke of it, its amazing how many other women will say they have that as well. I went to a bonfire party the other day in hat, scarf, polo neck, and boots, and while everyone else was freezing I was taking all the layers off because of at least six flushes that evening! So it can be of benefit at times. Don't let it get you down. I cannot take HRT due to blood clots, and I have psoriatic arthritis and take a lot of drugs for that, too. My rheumatologist saw me flushing the other day and told me to buy Flash Fighters from Holland and Barratt.

I did and they have eased quite a bit. Night sweats are the worse, quilt on, quilt off, window open, window shut, all night long! The more I talk about it to friends, the less a problem it seems to be.

I am 49 and have had menopause symptoms for three years, suffer night sweats and terrible hot flushes every day, I am tired, tetchy, have mood swings, cry loads, and, up until April this year, worked full time, I also have severe arthritis and suffer some days with that alone. In April, mum was diagnosed with cancer, and I sat at work and cried and cried, as I couldn't take any more, working, looking after mum, three men in the family home (they don't do much do they?), housework, cooking, etc. I think someone called my doctor and told him, and he called me. I visited his office and he signed me off work. It is now October, and I am still suffering all the problems of menopause, still suffering with the arthritis. Not having to work has taken a huge weight off my shoulders, as I get up in my own time in the morning, and if I don't want to face the world (let's face it, we don't have the time the way we feel), I don't have to. If I feel not too bad, I get up, shower, put my face on, and go and meet people. It's lovely to have that choice. Work really puts more pressure on you when you least need it. The only downside is I lost my salary, and we have had to cut back on loads of things. At first didn't think I could do it, but believe me six months down the line, I certainly wouldn't want to go back to work unless I felt well enough to do so (the arthritis is getting worse, so I can't see that happening).

I'm 47 and not on any hormone treatment yet but want to see my doctor as soon as possible, as I'm now suffering broken nights with sweating or just feeling like someone's set fire to me. I have irritable bowel and my symptoms have become much worse lately, so I feel lousy anyway. I'm tired, miserable, unsociable, and want to crawl away much of the time! I keep looking around at all these other women "of a certain age" and wondering how they're feeling and carrying on seemingly normally. I must be a very weak person! I work in a school, just part-time, but I couldn't manage more lately with working one-to-one with a child who has special needs. When I'm working, I'm working. I have to be there for him 100 percent, so there is no time for feeling exhausted or ill. How on earth do people carry on with their lives? If I could right now, I'd just stay at home all the time and never see anyone!

🗨 I am 55 and I have the night sweats. I am not talking about a little rush of redness, I lay on a towel because I am covered in sweat. I don't sleep well, I am always tired, bloated, have aching joints, heart palpitations, etc. I also work in a school and fortunately? (maybe) I am off work due to an injury at work. I had wrist surgery and am looking at back surgery. I only worked part-time, so somehow I would drag myself to work and get through the day. I also have fibromyalgia and IBS.
I wont take hormones, so I am just getting through it. I have cut back on caffeine, only having coffee in the morning, and I don't drink sodas. The last few weeks I have eliminated flour and sugar to maybe help a bit with the recent added weight. No one I know personally has the sweats like I do. They all fan themselves once in a while. Geez I would love to only have that. Actually I wish I had my periods again. I also now have osteoporosis. That was a shock.

🗨 I remember when my hot flashes started, they would fluctuate wildly and sometimes I would get about ten an hour, which would come very quickly and then just melt away. I think it was after about four to six months that they became more intense but less frequent. But to be honest, they changed all the time. Sometimes they very severe and other times I could just cope with them. I have been 18 months period free, and the flashes fooled me into thinking they'd gone for good about three months ago. I didn't have any for about three to four weeks, but guess what. They came back! I think these hot flashes are different for everyone in frequency, intensity, and how we all are able to handle them.

🗨 I had profuse sweating with hot flushes. I was having them on and off for a couple of years, which were reasonably bad, but I was coping until early last year. Then they got out of control, and day and night I would look like I had been in the swimming pool. Not a nice time, as it was very distressing. I went on Livial (Tibloene) in the end. This worked nicely for six or seven months, but then I started with the flushes and moods all over again. The flushes are not quite so bad (not as much the sweating) but still not nice, although the moods (deep sadness) and anxiety I think are worse. I found when I was having profuse sweating with the flushes, it was best to sit quietly and still and keep as calm as possible. Oh la la, that's easier said than done. It can make one very distressed.

Occasionally when I first wake up, I will get a peculiar feeling in my upper chest, kind of a flush without the heat, if you can imagine. It's a mildly tight, tingly feeling. I told the doctor about this a couple of years ago, and she ran the cardiac battery of stuff, so I'm pretty confident that my heart is okay. This happens only when I am first waking up, and it will happen for several days in a row and then disappear for days, weeks, or months even. It happened just this morning and that prompted me to do a search. I found that a symptom of hot flashes can be and "aura" or an odd feeling right before the flash. And I have sometimes noticed a hot flash right after the odd feeling. but I must say that my hot flashes are fairly mild and I might have missed noticing it at times after the odd feeling. Or maybe I got up and moved around and was distracted from noticing a mild flash. I have had off and on nausea for years. The only way to describe it was that I felt the same way I did when I was pregnant. I was sick to my stomach, but needed to eat. I would eat, feel better for a little while, then the nausea would come back. I went through every test under the sun and still my doctors cannot/will not attribute it to perimenopause. I wasn't thrilled about having all the tests done, but it did wonders for my peace of mind. I found this on another board and it has really helped for me: ginger zingiber officianale (500 mg,) one caplet three times a day, starting with first thing in the morning; licorice root extract (DGL) chewable tablets (it is vital to get DGL, as regular licorice can raise blood pressure) you chew one tablet twice a day. These taste pretty bad, but chase them with water and you should be okay. Both of these have helped me so much!

I get that weird shaky, jittery feeling after a hot flash and sometimes before. It's just like a bad case of low blood sugar, but eating doesn't help and I just try to go about my business until it passes. It does make me concerned about all these hormone shifts, etc. My poor body doesn't know what is going to happen next with all the shifts in hormone levels.

I'm 54. In November 2003 and August 2004, I had two major operations which triggered hot flashes. But once I had recovered from both, the flashes stopped, and at the time I didn't connect that they were hot flashes. I just thought I was weak from the operations and not able to control my body temp properly. I think my flashes started for real in about January 2005, and they were as many described here—very frequent, up to ten an hour at one stage. Then they stopped, then they started less frequently but more longer lasting and heat intensive. I also think it was around that time that my periods became less and less frequent. I'm now 14 months period free, and about a month hot flash free, so looking back I only had about two years of hot flashes, although it seemed much, much longer!

The hot flashes have tailed off. I wasn't sure at first if I was just coping better with them, or had got used to them, but there's a definite improvement, and I would say in the last week I've only had a couple. It was only yesterday I remarked to my husband that I'd not had one for three days. But I'm not holding my breath. I wouldn't be at all surprised if they start up again. I do still get anxious but am trying to be positive about that and work through it. Some days are worse than others. The only other change is that I've just had thrush. It's gone now, after taking a tablet and using cream, but I've only ever had that twice before in my entire life. I'm not currently taking any antibiotics, so I'm putting it down to this wonderful time of life!

I don't really suffer with hot flashes. When perimenopause first started, I did have some terrible night sweats, but never really had hot flashes during the day. I sometimes would get a small one, but nothing major. Now that I am fully in menopause, I don't have the shaky, cold, nauseous episodes very often. They only happen occasionally, but when it hits, it's pretty bad. I went to see an endocrinologist a while back and he said that it could be due to a hormonal surge. My hormones would take a sudden leap and my body would react with nausea and shakiness and feeling cold and clammy. I did not however experience any shortness of breath, but after an episode, I would feel really tired. I do think this could be a different reaction to hormonal changes than hot flashes.

I'm 48 and had night sweats when I was about 43. They lasted about six to eight months, then were gone. Now, the past two years I've had many of the other symptoms, but not the night sweats. Go figure! I think I may be just starting to get hot flashes, though I'm not sure yet. At work yesterday someone asked me if I felt okay because my face was red. Well, I was a bit warm. I just thought the heat was up too high. I looked in a mirror and boy, was my face red. Thinking back, I think I've been feeling this heat over the past two months. I just had my FSH levels checked this week and am waiting for results. I had them checked two years ago, but they weren't that high yet. My periods have changed a lot since then, so I'm thinking I may be closer now.

I'm 56 and started menopause at 53. I have never had a hot flash or night sweat. In fact, I too am cold most of the time. I asked my doctor about it because both my sisters had horrible hot flashes. He said not to worry and count my blessings. Some women just do not get them. I've always had a low body temperature and low blood pressure. I'm very healthy as far as I know.

I'm a 21-year old inhabiting a 53 year old overweight body (with a spare tire which would easily fit a tractor)! My confidence is at rock bottom, especially when my face lights up like a beacon, and I'm sure everyone in the room is staring. Since starting the menopause at 49, I just don't seem to have the incentive to be able to lose weight and keep it off. Each New Year I make the same resolution and am unable to stick to it. Apart from losing weight, my major ambition is just to get a good night's sleep. Hot flushes and the need to go to the loo (I have tested negative for diabetes) every two hours during the night make me exhausted during the day and it's back to the same cycle at night. I was prescribed Clonidine 25 mg. three times a day, yet this had no effect on the hot flushes. My doctor suggested I double the dose to six a day. I was like a zombie during the day, and there was no difference to the nights, so they are now in the bin! I am also taking Maca 500 mg. eight times a day. I originally got these to help with my lack of sex drive when a cup of tea and a good book are more exciting! I've been taking them for about three weeks but have not felt any effect on the sex drive or the hot flushes as yet.

I've just recently really started with the night sweats. Last night I was wearing a light summery type of nightgown and I woke up with my entire chest and under the breasts soaked with sweat. I get the hot flashes from time to time, and when I'm like that, I toss the covers off and then the next minute I'm freezing and have to cover up. No wonder we don't get a good night's sleep anymore. I am 49 going on 50 in two months. I have had no period now for going on seven months. And I don't miss the flow but hate all this other stuff that is going on.

I am 51 and still getting periods. Currently it has been gone for two months and my record for being without it was last year for four months. Anyway, I get cold flashes and not hot flashes. I guess I can say I got hot flashes in the form of the night sweats a couple years ago pretty regularly, but no hot flashes at all during the day or what other women describe. I've had a lot of other symptoms since my late forties, but not that. The cold flashes I imagine feel like the hot ones but in reverse. I get really cold, and even with two blankets it can be still where I feel chilled. It passes, but when it happens it is very uncomfortable.

I just thought I would share something I learned. I have had almost all perimenopause symptoms over the past year except hot flashes and some warm flushes. I am at the extreme end, chilled to the bone for hours at a time, which is all very upsetting. My thyroid tests are fine; however, I have been taking blood pressure medication for 16 years and recently discovered that this particular medicine I am on is also prescribed for women during menopause to stop hot flashes. Interesting! I had a jump start years ago without even knowing it.

I am 45. The power surges that I get usually start in my chest and wash over my whole body. It feels like someone shot a needle full of adrenaline into my system. I had one the other night that would come upon me and then subside, then five minutes later would come upon me again. This went on for 30 minutes. I have had anxiety attacks since I first started my period, but these don't feel like regular anxiety. I also get at times a squeezing feeling in my head at my temples. This sometimes is accompanied by my heart racing. It's weird. I would really like to find something that helps with this. I also get tingling in my hands and sometimes my forehead. My neurologist said that it could be part of my migraines. Do you ever get migraines with tingling? That might be what you are experiencing. I haven't heard about a link to blood pressure and tingling. You can get a big change in blood pressure when lying down. This sometimes happens to me. You may want to take your pressure when lying down then stand and take it to see the difference.

My periods have stopped completely. I am in menopause and haven't had a period for well over a year. My power surges usually happen in the morning, but I have had an occasional one at night. I would also sometimes get a queasy stomach along with the adrenaline rush. I can say that these episodes happen way less then they used to when perimenopause first kicked in. The way it was explained to me (by an endocrinologist) was that when your hormones take a severe dip is when the adrenaline-like surges happen. As your body adjusts to this new hormonal level, your symptoms fluctuate for a while, then level off, and you feel okay for a while. These hormonal adjustments can be severe at first and can happen quite frequently, but as you go along they happen less and less frequently and lessen in severity. The main thing is to try and remain calm when they happen, which is easier said than done, I know. I just really remind myself that it will pass, that it is just a hormonal fluctuation, and I'll be fine in a little while. Doing that helps to ease my anxiety and the episodes pass more quickly. I have read that as menopause approaches, some women do get heavier periods that are closer together. Mine was the opposite. My periods got lighter and lighter and less frequent until I stopped altogether.

I have never ever sweated like this in my life. I will be 48 in November and started this perimenopause when I was 44. It started slowly and then at 45 it pumped up by changing my period patterns. Then began the internal shakes and internal hot flushes. Anxiety and insomnia began, too. Now instead of getting the normal stinging chest and face, I am sweating profusely. At first I thought maybe this was a heart attack since this is one of the signs. But it's been happening for weeks, so I am thinking it's hormonal changes and sweating instead of having hot flashes like that burning sensation I used to get.

● I went through about six years of pretty bad hot flashes and night sweats. I started those symptoms just a year after having my uterus out at age 44 (the ovaries were kept). So yes, it can be difficult to pinpoint when it's all over if you don't have periods. I did go on Estradiol patch when the night sweats came every 22 minutes all night. My doctor felt I was probably at the end of menopause symptoms. I stayed on it less than a year. When I weaned off, I did get some mild symptoms back for a few months. Then I thought I was all set. But having no estrogen caused some problems for me. I knew vaginal dryness could be an issue, but I didn't know about vaginal atrophy, the horrible pain. I really had no idea how important it was to keep the vaginal tissues healthy. I started on the patch again this winter and, more importantly, the prescription vaginal cream. They made a big improvement with a couple weeks. Then I herniated my vagina because I don't have a uterus and because the pelvic floor and tissue weren't strong, it prolapsed. It was the most terrible thing to go through. I know that lack of estrogen can be a factor, adding another confusing factor. We are all different in how we react. At age 45, my mother went through menopause naturally and had no troubles at all. She has never taken anything and is now 76. I aged so much so fast with body and skin changes. I am 52 and have female health issues most women age 70 have.

● I am 42 and just starting year two of menopause. My symptoms a year ago were non-existent periods, bloating, weight gain, and night sweats. Never in my dreams did I expect to hear menopause. Not even perimenopause, but full blown. My doctor put me on birth control pills (Yasmine) that made an unbelievable difference. I lost the nine pounds I had gained within the first month or two. I also work out four to five times per week plus I work for Weight Watchers, so I am constantly watching what I eat, but nothing was taking off the weight. Anyway, I think my body must have gotten used to the pills because all of a sudden they weren't working anymore. All the old symptoms came back. So far, nothing is working. She switched my birth control to a higher estrogen, but it hasn't helped. I've also started to get "fever" flashes as opposed to hot flashes. I am at my wits end.

I have experienced the following, and only over the last three-fourths of a year or so (just turned 46 last October), in most severe order:

- Cold flashes, "clammy" feeling, only when at rest;

- Sleep disturbances (harder to fall and remain asleep), also waking more easily during the night (ready to throw my very loud, snoring boyfriend out!), and then having difficulty falling back to sleep (can't shut off my mind); and

- Period irregularities, with cycles running from short to long, slow start but heavier, and longer lasting at times, other times "normal," and mild PMS to none at all where I now just don't know what to expect from one period to the next.

- sleep disturbances, poor quality sleep, light sleep, insomnia

I am 50. I knew I would fall apart when I turned 50! I feel horrible. I have always been active. I ran or walked five miles daily. Now I can barely drag myself out of bed. I don't sleep well at night and wake up several times sweating and wet. I go to sleep, then wake up, then go back to sleep an hour or two later and sleep maybe a hour, then wake up again. This is almost every night. I also found out six months ago I have a small cyst on my right ovary. The doctor said I was in perimenopause for one thing and the cyst would go away on its own. Well, it still hurts. It bothers me so much that I don't feel like walking, and that is not like me. I have thought about using progesterone cream, but I am scared of it after reading the label that said it has been known to cause cancer. Also, I didn't know how the cyst would react to it. I am moody all the time and really hard on myself about the way I am acting. My whole body is changing and I just don't feel good.

I always get anxiety at night! It all stinks. I've also heard that fish oil helps. I take it, but I also take other things, so I don't know how effective it is. But it's worth a try if you are not already taking. I have fairly frequent insomnia (though not as bad as it used to be) usually around my period. Some nights I will only get three to four hours of sleep. I know if will feel terrible the next day, but I just push through knowing (or hoping) that I will be so tired that I will sleep the next night. Sometimes I'll just wake up at 4:00 a.m. for two or three days in a row. How annoying! I just accept it now as a part of my life.

I am not sure if my cycles are trying to start back up or not. I haven't had a period since June 2006. I have heard when we start perimenopause, some women continue to get their cycles and some don't. I seem to feel like I'm getting mine on occasion, but it never appears. The tiredness comes and goes. Tuesday night I was full of energy and dancing around my bedroom and then boom, I am tired the next day and am overly tired today, maybe because of an overactive dream I had and my honey had to wake me up from a dead sleep to get ready for work. At least he doesn't shake me awake but kisses me awake which is far more pleasant.

I have terrible nights at the moment, hot sweats, waking up every half hour, hardly getting any sleep, to the point I feel I would rather stay up. I am also having very strange dreams, and I feel it is the menopause, I keep having dreams of accidents and people being hurt. Only last night someone crashed their car, flew out of the window, and smashed their legs on the curb! Trouble is these dreams wake you up and the whole process starts again because you are hot you have to get up and freshen up, then you are wide awake! I am on steroids for arthritis, and a friend has told me it could be the steroids keeping me awake, but the dreams I am sure are the menopause. I used to get really weird dreams just before my periods years ago before I had a partial hysterectomy.

I think I can definitely say that when my hormones are really playing me up. I feel more anxious. If I wake up feeling anxious, then the first thing I think about is what I have to deal with on that day and where I have to go. I am totally aware of myself all the time and how I feel. It drives me mad.

💬 I feel bad that there are others who have panic and anxiety with this menopause thing, but at the same time it's comforting to know there are others out there who share this symptom. I also have considered Xanax. A friend has been on it for 15 years and started on it in her change. She is about 62 now, I am 55. I take Buspirone for anxiety now and it seems to work fine during the day; I feel my best between noon and about 8:00 o'clock at night and then all goes bad when it's time for bed. I dread going to bed at night, but I'm so tired I can't hardly hold myself up and yet I can't go to sleep once I lay down. My friend gave me a referral to see her doctor, because not every doctor will prescribe Xanax long term, but this one will. I'm afraid to switch doctors even though I don't like the one I have. It had definitely been the worst symptom for me. I'm 46 this year and came off the HRT after only five months because I think they were making my premenstruals worse. I can feel that the flushes have come back, but I am trying to go with it. I have been going through this for three years and missed a period a couple of months ago, so I hope I will start missing more from now on.

💬 I am 53 and my periods ended after a D&C two-and-a-half years ago. I've been feeling this type of exhaustion for quite a few years now. The doctor tested me for thyroid problems and anemia, and all tests came back negative. Sometimes, I think we try and run around as much as we did when we were many years younger, and it catches up with you. I can feel my exhaustion creeping up on me, and it's a weird feeling. I spent four months on HRT and felt a new lease of life (sleeping better and less tiredness), but my blood pressure kept going up, so I've had to stop taking it.

Urogenital atrophy, also known as vaginal atrophy (main article: Atrophic vaginitis)

- thinning of the membranes of the vulva, the vagina, the cervix, and also the outer urinary tract, along with considerable shrinking and loss in elasticity of all of the outer and inner genital areas

I am 52 and six years postmenopausal. I am experiencing extremely uncomfortable vaginal dryness. At my last gynecological exam less than a year ago, the doctor told me I was starting to experience vaginal atrophy. I have been sexually inactive for a little more than four years. I am on HRT, but I am weaning myself off the meds and am currently taking them five days a week. I'd like to try Replens. I know that there are two types--a gel packaged in single-use applicators, and a cream packaged with a reusable applicator.

I suffer from vaginal dryness, diagnosed as vaginal atrophy, for nine months. My life has been drastically altered as I wait to get better, if that's possible. There are times when I just sit at the edge of the bed with my face in a pillow and cry from the pain. It all started on New Year's Eve when I came down with a urinary tract infection. The infection went away but the pain stayed. I went through a number of painful tests and a cancer scare when my urine showed abnormal cells (atypical). A second test ruled out the atypical cells. My intent was to avoid use of any hormones at first, but I had to give in. I used Premarin cream for three weeks, and then I had to have my gallbladder removed. (Estrogen is known to cause gallstones in an already diseased gallbladder...that's me!) Then the dose was lowered, and I used a dab three times a week. After five weeks, I started to spot and had to go through a biopsy and polyp removal surgery. Then the doctor had me use Vagifem tablets, which I loved. The cream burned and this doesn't. But after using the two-week supply that he gave me and finally starting to get some relief, my insurance company refused to cover Vagifem to my great dismay. So back to cream. I'm now using Estrace cream three times a week, and it hurts a lot. But I'm trying to give it time to heal the thin tissue caused by lack of estrogen. I read that it takes anywhere from eight weeks to three months for estrogen to help. My insurance does cover the Estring but I just don't think I want that inside of me for three months at a time. And I already have pelvic pressure without an object in there! My symptoms are burning, pelvic pressure, urethral pain, and a feeling that I have to urinate all the time! It greatly altered my life, and my husband's! Very depressing. I feel so old at just 54 years of age.

- itching

Itching is one of the perimenopause symptoms. I have carried a tube of Benadryl cream in my purse for years. I'll start itching on my hand or foot or neck, always somewhere different. Sometimes I will notice little red bumps, other times it will just be the itching that bothers. I have no idea why it starts or stops. I hate it in the middle of the night, and then I can't go back to sleep. I think the itching comes from either an increase in allergies, dry skin, or loss of collagen in our skin due to changes in hormone levels. All I know is it drives me nuts some days!

I started menopause eight years ago, when I was 50. That was right about the time that I started getting hives over most of my body (except my face). I went to five different dermatologists who did blood tests, biopsies, etc. I also saw two allergists. No one could tell me why I got these hives that came and went. I suffered for nearly a year. My general practitioner told me that it could be from menopause (changes in hormones, etc.) and that the hives would eventually disappear. He was right. But it was so bothersome, I thought I would go crazy!

- dryness

I had a hysterectomy in 1994 and have been on HRT ever since. I will be 56 soon. This past January I started in with dryness, not so much vaginally but in the areas around it. The "lips" are so dry, they are chapped and painful. I am using hormone cream prescribed by my doctor three times a week. I also use a cortisone cream, Vaseline, hand lotion, and anything else I can get my hands on to get some relief. I can deal with the hot flashes and any other symptom of the change, but this dryness stuff is controlling my entire life.

- bleeding

Past 12 months have been a nightmare, as I have not had one normal cycle or period. I am nearly 47 years old. I can go from two weeks to eight weeks between periods, and sometimes I get spotting and slight bleeding for up to six weeks or I get incredibly heavy bleeding where I have to change a pad every hour and can feel that awful sensation of it pouring out of me. I had all the tests three months ago—hysteroscopy, D&C biopsy, and ultrasound—which were totally normal. So, I was diagnosed with dysfunctional uterine bleeding probably due to hormone imbalance. Due to family history of breast and ovarian cancer, I cannot do artificial hormones and my gynecologist can only offer me a hysterectomy, which I would happily have if I didn't have to have an operation and go into hospital and recover afterward. At end of September 2007, I went seven weeks with no bleed, then started spotting or slight bleeding. This lasted five weeks when I had ten very heavy days. Finally it just about stopped except for a tiny spot once a day. Two weeks later, I am into day three of a dreadfully heavy period. My doctor took blood tests to see if I need to supplement iron. Up to now, I have managed to keep my blood count normal, but I don't know how long that will last. I cannot take Tranexamic Acid to reduce bleeding, as it causes leg cramps, which could be a sign that I would be at risk of thrombosis. My gynecologist said if I get anemic, I seriously need to consider having a hysterectomy, but I am so terrified of hospitals and operations.

I'm 58 and about 18 months postmenopause I (had my last flow September 2005). I had some problems before that and had to have two D&Cs (one in February 2004 and one in March 2005). I think I'm finally done, but I do know I felt better when I was getting cycles. I had more energy and I slept better. Not sleeping for me is the worst part. I go right to sleep but then can wake up every hour on the hour! Not good when you are working full time and try to stay awake at work! Yes you can have "phantom periods" which are worse then the real thing. I did find out one thing though: If you go more than six months without a period and then get one, and especially if you go more than 12 months or a period lasts more than a week, it is worth a call to your doctor. They might want to check things out just to be sure. When I started skipping. I went four months and then had a "doosey" that lasted a month. I didn't think too much of it because I figured I had skipped and was just making up for lost time. In a week it came back again, so I called the doctor. I had to have some tests and then the D&C and I was told don't wait that long to call the doctor, especially if things are not normal. This is just such a "wonderful time of life." Not!

I've been going through perimenopause for a while. I use progesterone cream and take regular supplements. I also take Lexapro. For a couple of years my periods were very heavy and I'd get some spotting of the dark brown stuff a few days after it "ended" which was my body just cleaning out. The last two periods have been a little different and I'm just checking to see if anyone else has had this happen. I started my cycle on February 12 (26 days since last one) and I bled heavy for two days then very little for a couple of days. It seemed I stopped about the 15th. Then all of a sudden on the 18th, I went to the bathroom and there was more blood (like a regular flow). Then a little spotting yesterday and today, more blood, all kind of like a pause in my cycle.

I went for a bone density scan today and had a great chat with the menopause nurse there. She had experienced a relatively early onset of perimenopause at 39 and suffered for four years from perimenopause symptoms, including irregular bleeding and exhaustion, etc. She says it is very common in perimenopause but it's always best to check it out with the doctor as well, which I am doing at the moment (having hormone levels tested).

- watery discharge

- urinary frequency

I am 52 and still having major perimenopause suffering. Some days I wonder if I will live to the next day. As for the frequent urination, I am the queen of that! I get up numerous times during the night, every night. I take a low dose Ativan and a mild sleeping tablet each night, because I have to have some sleep since I work full-time. Since my stomach has always been my weak place, I have been suffering greatly with the all the perimenopause stomach issues, which increases my health anxiety. I, too, have searched the Internet about all these things, but have found that what I read makes everything worse. The blessing is that I have a new, wonderful doctor who really cares. He spent one-and-a-half hours with me on my first visit. I go for my pap on February 5, so I'll talk some more with him about all this suffering. I've gone two months without a period, so we'll see.

- urinary urgency

I'm 54 and almost through it, and I only had one very light period in the last 16 months. Like some women at about 49 or 50, my periods, which had always been regular as clockwork for years, suddenly started skipping a few months, then light and then heavy. I distinctly remember one morning, while sorting laundry actually, having a sudden urge to urinate, and worse, feeling I couldn't control it. This happened on and off for a few months, and I thought, heck I'm going to have to wear a pad all the time. Thankfully this eased off after a while, then virtually went away. Nowadays I'm fine during the day, but I have to get up a fair bit in the night. The last few months, I find after breakfast a bit of pressure building (which goes away). Could this be due to having a couple of glasses of juice and water?

- urinary incontinence

- increased susceptibility to inflammation and infection, for example vaginal candidiasis, and urinary tract infections

Skeletal

- osteopenia and the risk of osteoporosis gradually developing over time

- joint pain, muscle pain

I have been suffering from frozen shoulders this past year, and they have improved greatly but are still far from perfect. Some weeks they are pretty okay, and some weeks (like this week), I wake up with my arms stiff. Also, my hips seem to be so stiff when I wake up and also after sitting for a while. I am sick of it on top of all the other symptoms we have with menopause. Sometimes I think I am coming out of menopause (not with the stiffness though!) and then I fall back again. The tiredness is another thing. Right now I feel I could do with a nap.

I haven't had a period in a year. I am 49 and was on the pill and went off the pill in February. Here is my problem, and I don't know if this could be related to menopause: I have joint aches and pains all the time. I do not have hot flashes, I have no symptoms at all that I would be going though the change. I am not moody or anxious. I just ache all the time. I feel like I am falling apart.

The tightness in my calves, like someone was tying a rope around them, was the first huge symptom of perimenopause for me three years ago. At first my doctor thought it might be Peripheral Artery Disease, but since I didn't have any of the risk factors for that, he eventually realized it was perimenopause. I was sure I had heart disease, because I couldn't feel the pulse behind my knees, but it was just health anxiety. So, tightness it calves is a very real perimenopausal symptom!

My feet burn so badly it hurts to walk. Well, it just plain hurts all the time. I had this a year ago, and it eased up. But it is now back big time, with pain at a point of needing pain medications. At times my feet are very cold, then they get hot, and the pain feels like frostbite or when your hands get freezing cold outside and then you come inside and heat returns to them—it makes them hurt. It's awful.

Q My whole pelvic area hurts—everything down there. Also, I have a ton of bladder issues and no infection at the moment. I was told that the bladder has to heal, but this is ongoing. I'm using Vagifem once a week to help with frequency issues and urinary tract infections, although it may take weeks to feel the results. For the first two days after I use that, I have more pain down there. I understand that when everything is engorged with estrogen, it can cause pain and then settle down. I think I may be dealing with endometriosis, too. If the Vagifem doesn't work, I'm going on the pill. I really cannot take the pain in my pelvic area anymore. And I've had ultrasounds to rule out other stuff. Even a CT scan was done. But I'm certain this is all due to hormones.

- back pain

Skin, soft tissue

- breast atrophy

Q I am 46 years old and definitely perimenopausal. I've had a positive over-the-counter menopausal test as well, but I still have periods, although in the last ten months things are all over the place. I can go from three weeks to eight weeks between periods. I have always had ovulation pain, but now if I get it, it is agonizing for a week whereas it used to only last a couple of days. My periods are anything from three days to eight days long and some are short and light and others are long and very heavy. In the past I have rarely suffered from sore boobs, and if I did it was the week before my period and it only affects one boob and I get a very tender nipple. My last period was ten days late and was short and not heavy, but I had all the symptoms of ovulation on day six of my cycle! On day seven, I got my tender nipple. I have now had this for three days. I have had ultrasound and all is well down there! I realize that at this time of life anything goes, and I have had so many changes to my usual cycles, etc., that nothing surprises me. But I wonder how long I should leave it before I ask the doctor about my tender nipple. I would not even think about it if it had come at the usual time, but then I don't usually have ovulation on day six of my cycle either!

- skin thinning and becoming drier

During the period when my hormones were turning off and on like a light switch, I noticed that my normally oily skin turned dry when my hormones were off. Then the hormones would switch back on again, and my skin would be oily again. I have been on low dosage HRT for quite a few years, and my skin is less oily than it was, but not dry, except in the winter, perhaps from the lack of plumpness, I believe, a lack of collagen under the skin. This is what makes us look like we're not 20 years old anymore, regardless of how wrinkle-free our skin may be. Not that my skin is wrinkle free, mind you. But the plumpness is one of the main differences between young skin and uh, not-so-young skin. My hair has always been thick, that is, each hair is thick and I have a lot of it. What I am noticing is that it isn't so oily any more or probably it's that my scalp isn't so oily any more. I need more conditioner now. As for losing hair, I'm really only noticing that my pubic hair is pretty sparse now. Maybe if I weren't on hormones, I might notice hair thinning on the top of my head.

I dyed my hair about two months ago. I hadn't dyed it in over a year because my hair started to fall out due to low iron, stress, and a host of other reasons. I'm also in perimenopause. Right after this dye job (dark), I noticed all this hair falling. My sides got thinner, and it's like it took the new growth right out. It still falls, but it goes in spurts. Right before my period it seems to fall even more. What I want to know has anyone had success with getting their hair back after coloring it while in perimenopause? Or is this lost hair lost forever? I do see new growth at the top. I have lighter roots. But my sides feel so thin now. I'm never going to dye my hair again. I'm taking a lot of supplements in order to increase thickness, and every dermatologist and stylist tell me I have normal, healthy hair coming out of the top of my head.

- decreased elasticity of the skin

- formication, a sensation rather like pins and needles, more specifically like ants crawling on or under the skin

💬 I am 51 and still get my periods. However, they are changing somewhat. I have some hot feelings, but not flash-like symptoms. The strangest thing that has occurred most recently is this internal trembling feeling that first started at night but now is fairly constant throughout the day. It is bearable during the day, but it is awful at night. At first I thought it was my heart, but it's not. If I put my hand on my diaphragm area, I can feel the mild shaking all the time. It has progressed over the last few weeks into a constant internal sensation. I feel awful upon wakening (and every time I wake up throughout the night), and in the morning I am having anxiety attacks over this feeling. I am fearful that I have some awful disease and so I freak. This coupled with the muscle aches and spasms and the peculiar itchy crawly feeling under my skin has me freaking out a bit!

💬 It all started a year ago with the very heavy bleeding. I was afraid I was not going to be able to go out of the house. My husband had to bring me a change of clothes the first time. Last month after almost a year, the huge clotting has stopped. Now there are small clots. I did not go on anything. I refused to. I already take Lexaro and Ativan when needed. I was not going on something for the heavy bleeding. Now if the bleeding never had subsided, then that would have been different. But I would notice after a day or two of heavy bleeding it would stop and that was okay according to the doctor and normal at my age with changes in my body. But all the other symptoms are all still right there tucked away in my brain and body. My newest one is itching skin. My husband laughs every time I give a new symptom. Put me on some remote island and I will be fine.

Psychological

- mood disturbance

One day I am normal, and then the next day I turn into a maniac. It even seems like I feel funny driving sometimes. There are days also that I feel disoriented and just not myself. I don't have any hot flashes or sweats that are unbearable, really hardly any. Mine is all mental. I haven't had a period for over a year, so I'm over menopause, but feel worse than I did before. I am so afraid I have a tumor or something like that or I'm just actually losing my mind. I don't sleep right anymore, and I've been dieting and trying to work out. I also quit smoking, which has now been four months, so you'd think that my withdrawal and mood swing should be over from that. I just want to be okay again. I've posted over and over again, and everyone is probably getting sick of hearing this, but every time it comes back, it seems worse and I'm closer to losing it.

I get all kinds of strange symptoms. One minute I feel fine and the next I'm so cold or feel dizzy or my hands start to hurt, and I'm having breast tenderness. My underarm has been bothering me for a couple of months, which seems to be associated with PMS. I'm due for a mammogram, and my doctor will also do an ultrasound. He doesn't seem too concerned, so I assume that I shouldn't be too worried. He said it could be a side effect of some of the vitamins I take. I take a liquid multi that also has green foods. I stopped taking the vitamins three days ago to see if I feel any different. He didn't feel anything, so that put my mind at ease. Every day seems to be a new adventure. I do not drink or smoke or drink caffeine. I took up gum chewing, and it actually relieves some of the stress.

I am perimenopausal and am experiencing irregular cycles, sweats, now a form of cramping without a cycle, intense fatigue at 8:00 p.m. and awake all night. Worst of all I cannot seem to focus on anything. I am hoping that will pass but each day that continues, I panic something more is wrong with me.

Then I read your words and was reassured, thank goodness. Between low libido and "no mind," I am thankful I still exercise in the a.m., but then as the day progresses I seem to deteriorate. I keep waiting for the weeks that I will feel better to catch up on life. If this is the beginning of a long journey ahead, I need to seriously get an organizer and a foghorn to kick start me through the day. It is so awful, especially when you are a "go getter" and sitting listening to the breeze is the last thing I want to do at this stage in my life. I have had enough down time one week of the month, I don't need it consecutively.

I am now down to a three-day heavy bleeding period, and I have to change my tampon every two hours. But the worst is at night. I would never wear tampons to bed, but now I have to with an overnight pad. My mood swings are chronic and without warning, so my husband tells me. Being a sufferer of anxiety due to perimenopause, I often feel anti-social and disassociated from life. Sometimes forcing myself out into social places can be helpful as long as it isn't too far away from my comfort zone. I think we have been dealt a bad deck with all these changes, and as long as the doctors/gynecologists/cardiologists, etc., keep telling me that everything looks normal and I am not dying, I will tough it out the best way I know how with the best drugs available.

I am 51 and have brain fog. It's so embarrassing and makes me look stupid to others. I laugh it off and make up some excuse but it's really starting to get to me, things like forgetting what people tell me, going to get something and forgetting what I am looking for. I could even watch a movie and forget who died at the end. Now that is pretty bad. I also have had hot flashes on and off for almost ten years. Of course they have gotten worse the older I get. Mood swings are the worse. I can be irritable for a week or two and then out of nowhere, be in the greatest mood and happy for a few weeks. It's starting to affect my job, too. My boss who is a female is not at all sympathetic even though she is almost the same age. I was at risk of losing my job at one point.

I haven't been on the pill for about ten years or so. My periods started when I was 14. I have no children and had a termination of pregnancy in 1988. Last year my periods stopped for about nine months. They resumed again in January and February last year and have stopped again. At the moment I am experiencing some hot flushes and occasional insomnia. Currently I have no anxiety symptoms but have suffered periods of mild depression and anxiety since I turned 40. I am currently taking herbal menopause supplements. I am not sure if I am supposed to be or not since I am not officially menopausal (my periods haven't been absent for 12 months yet).

● After almost five years I'm now beginning to feel normal again although I'm still going through perimenopause. My periods are very irregular and last about three to four days. This journey has been a roller-coaster ride. I understand about not feeling normal and even sitting and pondering the big question, "What did I used to feel like before all of this began?" The depression, anxiety, panic attacks, de-realization, rapid mood swings. Do I need to continue? Yes, after five years I'm now beginning to feel more like myself. I still have those moments where previous symptoms appear, but thank goodness they are not lasting as long. To steal a cliché, I'm finally able to see the light at the end of the tunnel and it's not an on coming train!

● The anxiety is the worst! Five years ago at 47, I became extremely anxious about my health and thought something was terribly wrong with me. I was in and out of the hospital, and I even had my gallbladder removed. I thought I had pancreatic cancer. I have always been pretty much "together" before that time. My husband and kids were set back. I came out of that episode and, in the past five years, have had smaller episodes of anxiety. My hot flashes became nearly unbearable this past fall. I teach at a university and would be up in front of the class and suddenly sweat would be dripping down my back and on my upper lip, which was really disconcerting. So, in January 2007, I started taking the lowest dose of PremPro every other day. My mood improved overnight. I felt normal, but then I started having terrible lower back pain and I felt really bloated and very uncomfortable, so I stopped taking it on February 9. Now I am going through withdrawal I think. I am really anxious and jittery, have dizzy spells, my stomach is killing me, and I have all these health concerns back. I am a mess. I don't know if it can be attributed to the taking of hormone for a few weeks and then off, but probably. I'm not sure what to do. I am thinking about checking into bioidenticals at a very low dose. I keep thinking maybe I'm getting close to the end of menopause problems since it has been over five years.

Well, I was one of those who menopaused earlier at 43. It is indeed great. I just want you to know that you are not losing your mind and that's just how it feels during perimenopause. I never got mental health symptoms, but what happens physically can make you think you're imaging things. It's that shock of seeing our body change (like with me it was/is dark circles on and under eyes, some freckles, eyelashes straightening, osteoporosis, the worst part). So accepting that these changes are occurring is a difficult thing. And when one is in their early forties and experiencing it, it's a shock. Just do what I did when I was going through it and blame everything on the perimenopause. It turns out that most of it is indeed from changing. Have good discussions about everything with your gynecologist, though. He or she can reassure you. And at this time, if you are not completely satisfied with your gynecologist, change doctors. You should have excellent care during the time of your perimenopause.

I have experienced the following, and only over the last three-fourths of a year or so (just turned 46 last October), in most severe order:

- Cold flashes, "clammy" feeling, only when at rest;

- Sleep disturbances (harder to fall and remain asleep), also waking more easily during the night (ready to throw my very loud, snoring boyfriend out!), and then having difficulty falling back to sleep (can't shut off my mind); and

- Period irregularities, with cycles running from short to long, slow start but heavier, and longer lasting at times, other times "normal," and mild PMS to none at all where I now just don't know what to expect from one period to the next.

- irritability

- fatigue

I am 51 years old now. It seems like around the time I hit menopause (a bit early at 48), I just fell off a cliff health-wise. I started to develop high blood pressure, and then the hot flashes started. Sometimes I can't tell whether I'm having a hot flash or a blood pressure spike. For the first time in my life, I'm now taking daily medication for the high blood pressure. One of the side effects is fatigue, which makes me too tired to exercise every day, and that makes it harder to fend off menopausal weight gain. You get the picture. It becomes a vicious circle, one problem feeding off another. Less than a decade ago, I was running 5Ks in under 30 minutes. Now my knees are shot and I've developed chronic Achilles tendonitis. Then there are the "aesthetic" issues, such as thinning hair, my incredible shrinking lips, baggy skin around my caesarean scar. Menopause is a humbling experience! Previously and fortunately I was able to take good health and a sense of well-being for granted. Nowadays, sometimes for no apparent reason, I have bad days. I'm still having hot flashes (three years and counting). I'm hopeful that once all the hormones have settled down I'll be able to relax and make time for all the pursuits I didn't have time for when I was busy earning a living and raising a family. I just hope I'm still in one piece to enjoy it!

Well, my cardio doctor is trying something new on me. He thinks that my symptoms of dizziness and heavy fatigue may be due to my blood pressure dropping when I stand. I had a tilt table test and my heart rate increased when they stood me up. He put me on Florinef, a type of steroid, and I really don't want to take it but am trying it. I still have a lot of other symptoms due to perimenopause, such as anxiety, tingling in face, fingers and arms sometimes, panic attacks, stomach problems, and the list goes on. I hope that the medications I am taking don't just make things worse. I know that I am getting more anxious about the medications than I normally am during the day. I wish this menopause would end soon!

- memory loss, and problems with concentration

- depression and/or anxiety

🗨 I'm 48 and perimenopausal. Lately my anxiety level has skyrocketed. Out of the blue I'll start to feel anxious and then I have heart palpitations. The worst part is I've started to have odd thoughts—thoughts that make me feel bad and are nothing that I would have thought about three months ago. When I'm feeling good, it seems like my mind jumps back to the bad thoughts, just to bring me down. I feel like I'm trapped in this cycle. It might be something called Benign Fasciculation Syndrome or BFS for short. Maybe ask your doctor if that could be the explanation.

🗨 I am the queen of heart flutters. I have had skipped beats and fast heart rate episodes for years, ever since starting perimenopause. They have been fairly well controlled with a beta-blocker until the last several months. Now the flutters and skipped beats are there 24/7. I have started skipping periods, too, and I think these irregular beats are worse since missing periods. The only thing I can come up with is that my estrogen must be getting low and that is affecting my heart. I am so sick of these palpitations. I have tried upping my dose of the beta-blocker and I take more magnesium than usual. But the heart still flutters. I am about ready to start HRT and see if it helps. You might try taking magnesium and see if it helps you. Some women have really noticed a change after starting it.

🗨 Although I seem to be losing some of the horrible menopause symptoms (hopefully my body and mind are "settling down" to the hormone imbalance), I'm still battling with anxiety. I've got Tranx to take when needed, but when I do, my body still feels like it's in a state of "super tension." Sometimes I'm really knackered and just want to sit and relax and watch TV or something. I even find that hard, almost like I need constantly to be "up and doing" or "out and about." I don't know if this is because when I sit and try to relax and am not distracted, I begin to think about all the anxiety symptoms, which can kick them off again, or perhaps being alone. I'm pretty good at riding through anxiety most of the time, but it just seems so much more difficult if I try to relax. I've done all the usual relaxation techniques and breathing, and I know this takes time and effort. Sometimes it seems like nothing, but nothing I do will relieve this tension (exercise helps for a short time).

I am 46 and I started the first symptoms after I turned 40. Now the symptoms are getting worse. I was worrying a lot because I thought I had something bad. I started with dry skin really bad. I had to put on a lot of creams, and then my hair started falling out. I had the shakes, too. I feel like electricity going through my veins and muscles. Also, I had pain in my joints and now have pain on my left hip and waist. I went to the doctor. They did x-rays and nothing showed up. Also, I checked my heart and again everything was normal. I get a lot of panic attacks. My doctor wanted me to take Cymbalta, but I don't like to take medication. I want to take natural things. I just got some CDs to relax more. I want to start exercising. I don't know what to eat that will help me with this. I am glad that I am not alone. Also, another symptom I have is when I breathe, I smell something burning. It comes and goes. I think this is when I get panic attacks. I checked my lungs, too, and they are normal.

I'm 54. I've noticed over the last five years my head and pubic hair has thinned out quite a lot, not falling out, but just much thinner. To compensate for that, I have grown hair on my chin, upper lip, in my ears, up my nose and down my thighs! Mine is due to menopause, and if that's the cause of yours, then I don't think there's much you can do about it to be honest. I've been taking all the usual supplements (magnesium, calcium, fish oil, etc.) for about 18 months.

I'm 54 and 15-16 months without a period, so am officially postmenopausal. Probably eight to ten years ago, I started getting terribly itchy nipples, to the point that I wore out a few bras with the continual scratching and rubbing to ease the itch. They became painful because of the scratching to relieve the itch. Well, lo and behold, I grew hairs round my nipples, so I think for me it was the hair follicles starting to produce the hairs that made my nipples so itchy. The only things which gave any relief were moisturizer and wearing seamless bras, which I still do today. Great, isn't it, how hair thins from some places and starts growing in some other rather inappropriate places.

Q I am having PMS worse than I ever did before perimenopause. And I am not sure I can handle this! I have weird premenstrual spotting, mood swings, anxiety, acne flare-ups, hot flashes, and, new this month, the oh so enjoyable breast tenderness. I am 45 years old. When I was 40, my periods began to flow like a raging river for at least seven days a month. About two years ago, they began to slow down and now are only about three or four days long, not counting the premenstrual spotting. But I get this nasty PMS. I was very fortunate to have no acne problems, until now, and I feel like I am in high school again. The other night my son asked me if I had another eye, the zit was so huge. I never had PMS, my period was just something that came every 28 days and then left. The only time it was irregular was when I was pregnant with my children. I have never missed a day of school or work because of it. My cramping was minimal and really non-existent after the first day. I get totally paranoid regarding my health and everything else for that matter, send myself into an anxiety attack, and then realize my period should be starting within the next week. I feel like I am turning into one of those crazy women that you see on TV.

Q I've had this breakout about seven years, since my early forties. I get it mostly on my chin and neck area, and it flares up just before my period. I finally went to a dermatologist and have used various treatments, such as clindamycin, differin, and even an oral antibiotic. The antibiotic worked the best, but gave me a nasty yeast infection, so I had to stop it. That was back in September, and since then I've been pretty clear. I only need to use the topical once in a while. I don't know if the antibiotic knocked it out enough to get my system back to normal, or if it was going to stop anyway. I've just had FSH and LH tests to see if I'm closer to menopause, since my cycles have been changing. I don't have the results yet, but being close to actual menopause may be what's cleared me up a bit.

Q I am 52 pushing 53 and have had a problem with acne for about six years, since really starting into perimenopause. My face was great during teen years, but now the acne/rosacea is terrible. I don't really notice any age spots yet, but I am sure they are around the corner! I have had microderm abrasions and chemical peels, both from a dermatologist for the acne and acne scars. I didn't find either procedure very helpful. The peel goes deeper into the skin to remove top layers so new skin can surface. The peel is painful, and for a few days you look like you have been on the surface of the sun. The acne still came back, but some of the acne scars look a little lighter than before but not much. I had a series of four peels, every three to four months. The microderm abrasion makes your skin feel so soft, but that's about all it did for me, and there was no change in the acne scars or fine lines. My insurance wouldn't cover any of the procedures. They don't feel that acne is a medical condition, just a cosmetic problem. I would be interested in trying about anything. I hate leaving the house some days with the way my face looks.

I have been perimenopausal for a few years and hope I am almost through it. I do not get too any periods. I find that I get extreme morning "sadness" and, of recent, have been getting anxiety also. In fact I get all of a sudden any time during the day this wave of sadness just come over me for no reason at all. Maybe it is also part anxiety. I am finding that these days if I can force myself to take part in a couple of activities that I enjoy (or used to), and that is usually exercise for me, then I will feel better. Instituting it everyday is the hardest part. I went on Livial (tibolene) last July, as things were getting pretty bad, which helped a lot at first. But then in January I started getting hot flushes again and bad mood swings. I'm not sure whether it is worth staying on it now, as it doesn't seem to be doing the trick. And I have the fear of side effects, etc. Some days I find it hard to get out of the house. But it is much better to do so. Some gardening or exercise, etc., and seeing daylight also help with the mood swings. I can change my mind 50 times a day about what I really want to do!

I started getting acne in my forties (never had it as a teen). I finally went to a dermatologist and went through some different meds. The one that worked the best was an antibiotic, but it gave me yeast infections. My acne was definitely related to perimenopause. I'm 49 now, and it's cleared up a lot, although I still get the occasional acne cyst just before my periods (which I still get monthly). I had my FSH and LH levels tested earlier this year, and I'm closer to menopause than I was two years ago, so I'm thinking that's why the acne is getting better.

I have suffered with heart palpitations since my twenties. I have had high blood pressure, too, but my heart palpitations were from tachycardia. They found this out after I did a Holter Monitor test. That was many years ago. I just stopped taking my blood pressure medications because my blood pressure went so very low and we didn't know why. I know now, but it took a while to find out. Mine was caused to go so low because of my low vitamin D levels. It caused a host of problems for me. I told my gynecologist that I was having palpitations (usually normal for women who are in menopause), but she told me it's not normal if I'm on the estrogen patch and that palpitations are supposed to go away when you get on a hormone for menopause. She said that if mine continued, she'd have to further investigate it and I'd have to go off the hormone. I also think my palpitations were related to having GAD (General Anxiety Disorder) which I also was found to have about four years ago. These are not to be mixed up with panic attacks and other forms of anxiety. GAD is something one lives with all their lives, and I probably have had GAD since I was in my teens. It explains now why I behaved and why I felt the way I did at certain times. People with this disorder are chronic worriers and this affects your entire system, especially your nervous system because the "fight or flight response" is on constant go, which affects your entire nervous system. I'd wake up as early as 3:00 a.m. and want to get up. By the time 2:00 p.m. rolled around, I'd felt like I had been up for days. It affected my life and my sleep cycle. I was constantly agitated and would snap at my family when asked a simple question. I was ready to fight with people on the phone at work or my coworkers if they said something that irritated me. I couldn't let things go if someone said something to me that insulted me. I'd carry it with me for hours afterward and bring it home with me only to ponder it the next morning when I'd wake up. I was getting sicker and sicker by the moment. I've heard that people with this disorder also feel things more, physically that is. They put me on an antidepressant, which also was an anti-anxiety medication. I am now on Zoloft, and wish I had not fought my doctor to take medication all those years before. It saved my life. I began to see things open up and things didn't seem to be so negative in my life and there was finally answers and hope to my problems. I began to have energy again, and I was able to sleep past 3:00 a.m. My heart palpitations came to a halt. I had to stop having full brewed coffee and switched to instant coffee because there's less caffeine in it. I add more water to my cups of coffee so I can have the pleasure of having my coffee and not have it give me the effects of just having done an amphetamine. I'd bounce off the walls and want to crawl out of my skin when I drank full brewed coffee.

I've had blood pressure (BP) problems since starting perimenopause a few years ago. However, it seems to be a transient problem. I take my own BP everyday. Occasionally it went into the upper limits (or lower) of stage 1 hypertension and stay that way a couple of days. About 30 percent of the time it would be in the lower limits of stage 1. The calcium/magnesium supplements seem to keep it in check, and now I usually don't measure in the stage 1. Also, now I kind of know what foods bother my blood pressure and I can stay away from them. I keep track of everything I eat everyday and I've learned quite a bit about what my body will and will not tolerate. The remaining unsolved problem with blood pressure is that sometimes vitamins, herbs, or medicines make my blood pressure go up, so I wind up not taking them. I never take a lot of anything. Every time I tell a doctor or the person in the vitamin store, all they say is "that shouldn't happen." Or, they'll try to tell me that it's not happening, which really ticks me off.

I'm 43. I missed three periods last year and assumed I was perimenopausal; however I stopped taking the antidepressant medication I was using and my periods returned as normal. I have recently started to take the same medication again and missed one period though the next one came on time. I just don't know whether I'm ovulating less and my periods are erratic due to perimenopause or whether it is the medication! My doctor seems to think the meds can't cause this. I don't have hot flushes, I do have terrible mood swings, I am not overweight but can't lose weight, my tummy swells, and I feel like I have permanent PMS.

Losing weight and diet were changed for the better when I took a year's worth of college lifting classes to lose the pounds when I turned 50. My energy went up and gone was the fuzzy thinking, feeling off balance or dizziness after starting this, especially the blues. But I never had much problem with this to begin with. I always did find positive ways to recover from depression. The lifting helps keep the pituitary gland producing HGH closer to levels when you are young. Muscle weakness went away as I built it up to increase strength. One added bonus from menopause though is that I no longer get the achy flare-ups just before and during my periods and my face has been clear for years now.

I am going through a period of severe anxiety again. This has happened on and off for five years or so. Last week I was having these dizzy spells, and these escalated into my thinking I must have a brain tumor or something. I had a CT scan on Friday and everything was normal, but I am in a real tough spot right now. I get up in the morning and I feel so jittery and anxious, my stomach is bothering me, and it feels full of acid. I am a mess. I started taking PremPro in January and felt great emotionally, but I started having cramps and bloating and pain so I quit taking it. That was a month ago. I am wondering if I set things back and now am dealing with this anxiety. I have been thinking about some other form of hormone replacement like Estrace with some type of progesterone, as I still have all my parts.

I had a complete hysterectomy in 1989, when I was only 39 years old. It was the worst nightmare of my life. It took me ten years to feel like myself again. I had everything described here, but more. The depression and fatigue were so bad, I thought I just can't live the rest of my life feeling like that. I thought it would never end. I felt like I had jet lag, I spaced out, I walked around in circles, not knowing what to do, and I thought I was going crazy. I started to get obsessive, sweeping the floor over and over. My heart would feel like it was jumping out of my chest. I couldn't sleep for years. I felt like my body was buzzing like an engine that wouldn't shut off. I would wake up in a cold sweat, dripping wet, then would get a chill. I went to doctor after doctor, and they all said the same thing: "You are getting your estrogen, you shouldn't have these complaints, it's all in your mind, you need see a shrink." I felt so alone. I finally found a doctor who took my estrogen levels and said they were quite low. He pumped me up with injections of estrogen for about four months. Slowly, and I mean slowly, each year it would get a little better. The fatigue and depression started to lift. And then I was sleeping better, and so on. You probably will not go through what I did, because you are going through a natural menopause, not surgical. It will take time, you're not going crazy, all the things you are experiencing are not in your head; it's the body going through withdrawals from estrogen. Imagine if you were a drug addict and had to go cold turkey, that is what is happening, you are getting estrogen withdrawal.

I have the stupid spare tire that just started accumulating on my mid-section over the past couple of years. I feel like I am walking or sitting with a stupid inner tube strapped around my waist like the ones we use for the kids or someone who can't swim. It seems to want to get into the way of everything. It pushes up and makes it harder to get a lungful of air. I have terrible indigestion (at least I think that is what it is). I feel like I have a ball sitting in my belly just under the sternum and I get a wicked pressure in my chest from time to time. I get dizzy spells on occasion or just a loss of balance and feel like my entire head is radiating some sort of heat and I get itchy. Today I am just feeling blah and as if I am in a total fog. My eyes especially are extremely tired. I feel like I could easily climb into bed and go fast to sleep. That is probably what I need to do but since I'm working I can't. I've never felt this crappy in my life. Why is it that when we turn of a certain age we seem to just start falling apart? I am going to be turning 50 in March and I thought at first that this milestone wouldn't bother me, but it's starting to. I get the anxiety attacks even when I don't feel like there is anything to be anxious about. Thoughts of death and cancer and all that gobbledygook and I lay in bed at night and try to use breathing exercises to calm myself down. My heart races or palpitates and I feel like my entire inner body is vibrating. I can't just relax. Every single muscle in me is tense. I hate this.

I am sure anxiety makes the symptoms of the menopause much worse. I have often heard that people who are more relaxed don't seem to have such a hard time dealing with the menopause. I have no personal experience of Effexor, although I do know a few people that have taken it for depression/anxiety. The one thing common thing I have heard from the people taking it is that although it worked for them, it was a very hard medication to wean off. I also always try to eat well, etc., although I don't really exercise as much as I should. I would agree though that people really have no idea what we go through with mood swings and hot flashes, etc. My partner laughs when I have a hot flush, as he thinks it's amusing that my face suddenly goes all shiny and I get all flustered with it.

My symptoms occurred at two four-week intervals over the past two years. However, the feeling of doom and gloom and extreme anxiety is ever present, along with dizziness, anxiety/depression, bouts of terrible indigestion and difficulty swallowing, muscle aches and pains (behind my shoulder blades, in my breast bone, and in my arms, knees, and legs), extreme fatigue at times like the flu, crying (so bad I can't stop) at everything, intense worry over everything, irritable bladder about once a month, irritable bowel, itchy/burning/crawling skin, hot flashes, night sweats, sleepless nights, heart flutters when just resting, loss of sexual drive, nausea, and indigestion with belching. Two years ago, I felt great. I could walk miles and move and lift anything. Now, I can barely get up from lying on the floor.

Sexual

- decreased libido

I have been having just about every perimenopause symptom under the sun for about four years. I'm now 45. One that hasn't hit me yet is lack of libido. In fact, mine seems to have gone the other way. But after having sex, I have a heavy feeling of anxiety that can last for quite awhile, sort of like everything getting revved up and then afterward having an extreme feeling of anxiety and nervousness. I've never had this type of feeling after sex. I swear I've felt better with all the other symptoms when I just didn't have sex at all, but I hate to give up that part of my life. But, it's like it gets something going hormonally.

I'm 43 and, after having my little girl at the age of 40, my periods stopped. I went to the doctor and had a blood test. I was told that I am going through premenopause. And that's when the problems started—hot flushes every 15 minutes, depression, changes in libido, and a hundred other things. It is having an effect on my family, especially my partner, and I would really like to solve this once and for all. But I don't know how.

I'm 39 with four children. My mother and sister both started menopause at this age. For the past ten months, I've had no sex drive at all. It's driving me crazy. I went to doctors, and all they came up with was "stress." I can't go by missed periods because I'm on the Depo shot, and I don't get periods then. Also, I have experienced some hot flashes in the past, but I thought them to be related to anxiety.

- vaginal dryness and vaginal atrophy

Here is my story and a description of what happened to me three years ago. I was 47 and doing great! I exercised, ate right, but started having super heavy periods. One day at work, during a heavy period, I had a gusher. As I was walking to my office, all of a sudden my right arm tingled, and a sensation shot up into my arm, which led to my neck and then my face. My right side (arm on up) was locked up and my right side of my face pulled over to the left side. I could not talk, and outward appearances were of a stroke. I could process information, did not faint, and could nod my head in answer to questions. This only lasted less than a minute, I could feel the sensation leaving my face and arm, and was fine right after. My doctors (two specialists) said seizure, one doctor said mini-stroke. They put me on so much medicine and made changes, such as Celexa to Prozac, to Paxil, to Buspar. I was losing myself and hated how I felt, so I took control. After two months of knowing I was headed down the wrong road, I went off the medications and started meditating. My faith strengthened as well. I became happier. I still deal with the above issues daily, but try to have a good sense of humor to help me deal with it. Bottom line, the doctors were using anxiety medicine to treat whatever happened to me. Turns out, after lots of testing, I am hypoglycemic which can, when the stars are lined up right, lead to a seizure when combined with my intake of high energy drinks a couple of times a day (tired all the time, another indicator of the big menopause) and lots of coffee. No wonder I had a seizure! Who wouldn't? My doctor says my bladder, front of my vagina, and my uterus have all fallen. So he wants to remove my uterus and lift and secure my vagina and bladder with, you guessed it, a hammock! (Why do I get the image of my bladder lounging around on a warm beach in a hammock between two palm trees?) And he has prescribed Provera for bleeding control in the meantime so I won't have so much clotting. After researching this drug, I am thinking no way!

- problems reaching orgasm

- dyspareunia or painful intercourse

One cohort study found that menopause was associated with hot flashes; joint pain and muscle pain; and depressed mood.[6] In the same study, it appeared that menopause was not associated with poor sleep, decreased libido, and vaginal dryness.[6]

Need for more education about menopause

Many women arrive at their menopause years without knowing anything about what they might expect, or when or how the process might happen, and how long it might take. Very often a woman has not been informed in any way about this stage of life by her physician or by her social group. In the USA at least, there appears to be a lingering taboo which hangs over this subject. As a result, a woman who happens to undergo a strong perimenopause with a large number of different symptoms, may become confused and anxious, fearing that something abnormal is happening to her. There is a strong need for more information and more education on this subject. [5]

At the age of 39, I started obvious perimenopause symptoms—irregular periods, dry skin and vagina, as well as night sweats during the "off" hormonal times, followed by normal periods and moisture during the "on" times. I suspect that it took another ten years for me to be considered officially menopausal, as it took that long for the low dosage to become insufficient to combat the symptoms. I figured at the time that I had just used up my allotment of hormones early because I had regular periods every 23-25 days for my entire reproductive period (with 15 periods per year instead of the normal 12-13), and I didn't have any children. This may be an entirely bogus speculation on my part, but it helped me accept that I was just in the early half (before 50) rather than the late half (after 50) to reach menopause. Cysts can, I understand, affect the hormones. It is appropriate to research further and see if there are any underlying causes that can be treated.

I'm 48 and have been postmenopausal for eight years. I went through menopause really quickly and early. I've been reading about "PTLS" (Post-Tubal Ligation Syndrome)) which can be a very real cause for early menopause. I was amazed to find out that many women have suffered the symptoms of PTLS after having a tubal ligation. I had mine when I was 38 and within two years was totally menopausal much to my dismay. It seems when they cut/burn/tie your fallopian tubes during the TL procedure, it cuts off the much needed blood supply to the ovaries and, in some women, can result in menopausal symptoms. No wonder! I suffered all the symptoms of menopause before my time, thanks to this procedure and doctors not informing me of such. Many women are having TL reversals because of this and are finding that it "cures" all the menopausal and many other ill causes from TL. I wish I had known.

I'm 46 and am in perimenopause at the moment. This is actually my second menopause. My first one happened when I was in my late twenties. I stopped ovulating and menstruating and my hormone levels went through the floor—all except for my testosterone. All women have testosterone, just much lower levels than men. Mine at that point were at the lower levels for a man. What I was finally diagnosed with was something called Polycystic Ovarian Syndrome. (PCOS) It is a syndrome that most women who are having fertility problems are diagnosed with. I had already had my daughter by then, and we were not trying to get pregnant, but I was just concerned why everything had stopped. Cysts can produce hormones and they can also cause other hormones to fluctuate up or down. The usual treatment for it is to introduce additional hormones, such as estrogen and progesterone. There is also frequently a tendency for insulin resistance with PCOS, and so many women are put on diabetic medications. Some women have some of the symptoms and some have all of them. The one constant is multiple cysts on one or both ovaries. These are always simple cysts (benign). In my late thirties, completely out of the blue, my normal cycle began again. I had not had any treatments for over six years! Even my gynecologist had no idea why it all changed. Now I'm in perimenopause, so I get to go through this all over again.

I'm now in menopause at 45, and I have seizures. Back when I was four, I started having seizures that lasted until I was about ten when they stopped. In September of 2006, when I was close to menopause, I started having seizures once in a while, which were not bad. Now I'm in menopause and am still not on any medications for seizures. I have a seizure about once or twice a week, and sometimes I can go as long as a month before I have another. I had also been misdiagnosed as having panic when it was really a seizure. I, too, am scared to leave the house. Some days I do fine and other days I don't. I believe hormones have a great deal to do with my seizures because I went from way back when I was four to ten and then here I am 45, having seizures again. Also, I have a family history of seizures. Scans show nothing, but my doctor said sometimes he just has to go by symptoms. I had a big seizure on December 4, another one on December 6, and another one on December 14. The one on December 4 was witnessed by my sister who wrote a paper of what she saw. I'm taking it to my doctor to show him I was out cold that day and still don't remember anything except going to my mom's and seeing my sister's white sweater. I can't say for sure if menopause triggers seizures, but I have heard they do. It seems strange that I'm in menopause due to early menopause because of surgery and I'm having seizures now, so I'd say yes, most likely, and they are scary. With a seizure, I just drop to the floor and lay there—I don't hyperventilate, and its like I'm sleeping. But with panic, I freak out and start breathing heavy. It feels like I can't breathe and I start crying. When I have a seizure, my eyes flicker, so to me menopause plays a role. I also used to suffer with PMS but never had a seizure. I cried a lot from my seizures, but I just assumed it was my menopause. While on HRT, my crying and depression have gone away so far. Still, I cry every time I have a seizure. I hate living with them. I'm due to have another MRI. I was supposed to in August, but my regular doctor would not give me anything to calm me down. He said he doesn't believe in Xanax or stuff like that, but I take Xanax now for panic. I do have both panic and seizures, and the HRT seems to be helping me a great deal. I won't ever go completely without them. They gave me back my life. When I get on the seizure medications, I will be the person I was before 2006.

Treatment

Perimenopause is a natural stage of life, not a disease or a disorder, and therefore it does not automatically require any kind of treatment. However when the bodily effects of perimenopause are severe and disruptive, they may be alleviated through medical treatments.

Hormone therapy, also known as hormone replacement therapy

See also *Hormone replacement therapy (menopause).*

There are several types of hormone therapies, with various possible side effects. Hormone replacement therapy or HRT, known in Britain as Hormone Therapy or HT, and the SSRIs appear to provide the most reliable pharmaceutical relief. However, adverse effects of one kind of HRT (equine estrogen combined with a synthetic progestin) are now well documented. See the section below on "Adverse effects of conjugated equine estrogens".

In addition to relief from hot flashes, hormone therapy remains an effective treatment for osteoporosis.

A woman and her doctor should carefully review her situation, her complaints and her relative risk before determining whether the benefits of HT/HRT or other therapies outweigh the risks. Until more becomes understood about the possible risks, women who elect to use hormone replacement therapy are generally well advised to take the lowest effective dose of hormones for the shortest period possible, and to question their doctors as to whether certain forms might pose fewer dangers of clots or cancer than others.

Alternative dietary supplements for treatment of menopause symptoms afford anywhere from significant to moderate relief of these symptoms. Some botanical sources, referred to as phytoestrogens, are known to have an estrogenic effect on the body and therefore create a moderated estrogenic effect. Others, such as femarelle, were found to have Selective Estrogen

Receptor Modulator (SERM) qualities [7], thereby reducing the safety risks involved in estrogenic-like treatments.

In HT or HRT, one or more estrogens, usually in combination with progesterone (and sometimes testosterone) are administered, not only to partially compensate for the body's loss of these hormones, but also in an attempt to keep the levels of these hormones in the body much more consistent than they are naturally in perimenopause.

In those women who have no uterus (usually due to a previous hysterectomy) estrogen alone is a suitable hormone therapy. Women who still have a uterus need to take progesterone in addition to estrogen, in order to ensure that the endometrium, the lining of the uterus, does not build up too much, which would be a risk for cancer of the endometrium.

Conjugated equine estrogens

See also *Types of Hormone Replacement Therapy.*

Conjugated equine estrogens contain estrogen molecules conjugated to hydrophilic side groups (e.g. sulfate) and are produced from the urine of pregnant Equidae (horses) mares. Premarin is the prime example of this, either alone or in Prempro, where it is combined with a synthetic progestin, medroxyprogesterone acetate. However Premarin, and especially Prempro, are associated with serious health risks.[8]

In January 2003, the U.S. FDA required Wyeth to affix a "black box" warning to PremPro, stating:

"WARNING: Estrogens and progestins should not be used for the prevention of cardiovascular disease. The Women's Health Initiative (WHI) reported increased risks of myocardial infarction, stroke, invasive breast cancer, pulmonary emboli, and deep vein thrombosis in postmenopausal women during 5 years of treatment with conjugated equine estrogens (0.625 mg) combined with medroxyprogesterone acetate (2.5 mg) relative to placebo (see Clinical Pharmacology, Clinical Studies). Other doses of conjugated estrogens and medroxyprogesterone acetate, and other combinations of estrogens and progestins were not studied in the WHI ..."

Adverse effects of conjugated equine estrogens

See also *Types of Hormone Replacement Therapy*.

Women had been advised for many years by numerous doctors and drug company marketing efforts (at least in the USA) that hormone therapy with conjugated equine estrogens after menopause might reduce their risk of heart disease and prevent various aspects of aging. However, a large, randomized, controlled trial (the Women's Health Initiative) found that women undergoing HT or HRT with conjugated equine estrogens (Premarin), whether or not used in combination with a synthetic progestin (Premarin plus Provera, known as PremPro), had an increased risk of breast cancer, heart disease, stroke, and Alzheimer's disease. Although this increase in risk was small overall, it passed the thresholds that had been established by the researchers in advance as sufficient to ethically require stopping the study.

When these results were first reported in 2002, the popular media sensationalized the story and exaggerated the risk, while the manufacturer continued to attempt to minimize the degree of risk. However most news stories failed to mention that the average age of the women in WHI was 62 years old, significantly older than the time when most doctors start patients on HRT, and in fact many years into postmenopause. In order to enroll in the study, patients had to be asymptomatic of hot flashes, so they would not know whether they received the placebo. For these reasons WHI was not representative of generally accepted clinical practice.

The 2002 and 2003 announcements of the Women's Health Initiative of the American National Institute of Health and The Million Women Study of the UK Cancer Research and National Health Service collaboration respectively, that HRT treatment coincides with a increased incidence of breast cancer, heart attacks and strokes, lead to a sharp decline in HRT prescription throughout the world [9][10][11], which was followed by a decrease in breast cancer incidence [12][13][14].

On hearing the news about the WHI study, many women discontinued equine estrogens altogether, with or without their doctor's approval. The number of prescriptions written for Premarin and PremPro in the United States dropped within a year almost to half of their previous level. This sharp drop in usage was followed by large and successively larger drops in new breast cancer diagnoses, at six months, one year, and 18 months after the drop in Premarin and PremPro prescriptions, for a cumulative 15% drop by the end of 2003. However, the apparent meaning of this correlation is called into question by the fact that prescriptions of PremPro and Premarin fell dramatically in Canada as well, but no similarly dramatic drop in Canada's breast cancer rates was observed during the same time period. Studies designed to track the further progression of this trend after 2003 are under way, as well as studies designed to quantify how much of the drop was related to the reduced use of HT/HRT.

Other forms of hormone therapy

See also *Types of Hormone Replacement Therapy.*

The adverse biological effects of xenoestrogens and progestins revealed by studies of Premarin and PremPro do not necessarily generalize to supplementation with human forms of estrogen and progesterone. For example, a pilot study reported in JAMA by Smith, Heckbert, et al.[15] found clinical evidence that oral conjugated equine estrogens caused clotting, but the other estrogen compound tested in the same study, bioidentical esterified estrogens, did not. Conjugated equine estrogens were found to be associated with increased venous thrombotic risk. In sharp contrast, the study found that users of esterified estrogen had no increase in venous thrombotic risk.

Due to the controversy about Premarin-based hormone therapy, a number of doctors are now moving patients who request hormone therapy to help them through perimenopause, to bioidentical hormone products.

Estrace is a form of the precursor to estrogen in the human body known as estradiol, which products have produced fewer side effects than conjugated equine estrogens[16]. Prometrium is a bioidentical progesterone which can be used in conjunction with Estrace.

However, all hormone replacement therapies probably do carry some health risks, including high blood pressure, blood clots, and increased risks of breast and uterine cancers. Women who have had a hysterectomy seem to tolerate estrogen-only therapy with fewer risks than apply to mixed-hormone therapy in women who still have a uterus.

The anti-seizure medication gabapentin (Neurontin) seems to be second only to HRT in relieving hot flashes.[17]

Selective Estrogen Receptor Modulator's (SERM's)

SERM's are a category of drugs, either synthetically produced or derived from a botanical source (Phytoserms), that act selectively as agonists or antagonists on the estrogen receptors throughout the body. While most SERM's are known to increase hot flushes, Femarelle (DT56a) decreases them[18][19]. In addition to the relieving effects on menopausal symptoms, Femarelle also increases bone mass density (BMD) [20], making it protective against osteoporotic fractures. These effects are achieved by an agonistic interaction with estrogen receptors in the brain and bone. On the other hand, an antagonist interaction with estrogen receptors in the breast [21] and uterus[22] [23], has no effect on these tissues.

Antidepressants

Antidepressants such as paroxetine (Paxil), Fluoxetine hydrochloride (Prozac), and Venlafaxine hydrochloride (Effexor) have been used with some success in the treatment of hot flashes, improving sleep, mood, and quality of life. There is a theoretical reason why SSRI antidepressants might help with memory problems—they increase circulating levels of the neurotransmitter serotonin in the brain and restore hippocampal function. Prozac has been repackaged as Sarafem and is approved and prescribed for premenstrual dysphoric disorder (PMDD), a mood disorder often exacerbated during perimenopause and early menopause. PMDD has been found by PET scans to be accompanied by a sharp drop in serotonin in the brain and to respond quickly and powerfully to SSRIs.

Blood pressure medicines

About as effective as antidepressants for hot flashes, but without the other mind and mood benefits of antidepressants, are blood pressure medicines including clonidine (Catapres). These drugs may merit special consideration by women suffering both from high blood pressure and hot flashes.

Complementary and alternative therapies

Medical non-hormone treatments provide less than complete relief, and each has side effects.

In the area of complementary and alternative therapies, acupuncture treatment is promising. There are some studies indicating positive effects, especially on hot flashes [24][25][26] but also others [27] showing no positive effects of acupuncture regarding menopause.

There are claims that soy isoflavones are beneficial concerning menopause. However, one study [28] indicated that soy isoflavones did not improve or appreciably affect cognitive functioning in post-menopausal women.

Other remedies which in some studies appear to work well, but in other studies appear to be no better than a placebo include red clover isoflavone extracts and black cohosh. Black cohosh can cause the stimulation of pre-existing breast cancer.

Other therapies

- Lack of lubrication is a common problem during and after perimenopause.[29]Vaginal moisturizers such as

Replens can help women with thinning vaginal tissue or dryness, and lubricants such as K-Y Jelly or Astroglide, can help with lubrication difficulties that may be present during intercourse. It is worth pointing out that moisturizers and lubricants are different products for different issues: some women feel unpleasantly dry all of the time apart from during sex, and they may do better with moisturizers all of the time. Those who need only lubricants are fine just using the lubrication products during intercourse.

- Low-dose prescription vaginal estrogen products such as Estrace cream or the Estring are generally a safe way to use estrogen topically, in order to help vaginal thinning and dryness problems (see vaginal atrophy) while only minimally increasing the levels of estrogen in the bloodstream.
- In terms of managing hot flashes, lifestyle measures, such as drinking cold liquids, staying in cool rooms, using fans, removing excess clothing layers when a hot flash strikes, and avoiding hot flash triggers such as hot drinks, spicy foods, etc, may partially supplement (or even obviate) the use of medications for some women.
- Individual counseling or support groups can sometimes be helpful to handle sad, depressed, anxious or confused feelings women may be having as they pass through what can be for some a very challenging transition time.

Treatment Options

My doctor asked if I wanted him to prescribe something and I said yes. He prescribed Ativan (half a pill at bedtime when needed) for the anxiety and Celebrex (one or two per day) for the muscle pain. Well I went to the pharmacy and got the Ativan, but the Celebrex was $150! I asked them why so much, and they said because it is not formulary anymore due to the lawsuits. Hmmm. That didn't sound good. I told them that I would have to wait on that one until I called my insurance company and did some research on it before I would take it. The pharmacist actually told me that I would be better off taking 400-600 mg. of Motrin every six hours. He said there really isn't any difference between the two.

I use the naturally compounded progesterone cream on days 10 to 25 of my cycle, counting day 1 the first day of my period. If you haven't had a period for a while, I was told by my doctor to just pick a day and start using it. You might spot a little during this time, but just keep using it unless you start a full-blown period, then stop using it and begin your count. The cream has helped with all of my symptoms tremendously. I also read somewhere that if you have a heavy period, you can rub a little of the cream on your stomach a couple times a day, and it helps to lessen the flow. I also take calcium, magnesium, and flax seed oil capsules. This combination seems to work really well. I don't take a multi vitamin, because vitamins make me nauseous, so I just try to eat really healthy food me with an occasional junk food binge, which I end up paying for the next day!

I find it beneficial to take calcium and magnesium an hour before going to bed to help me rest. Lately, I've been experimenting with 1,300 mg. primrose oil with my breakfast, and it has helped with my mood, spacey feeling, and overall well-being. I've also noticed that the liquid flaxseed oil helps minimize the pain I've been having in my left knees for several years. I also take prescription medication, so it's best to not mix them with the primrose and flaxseed oil.

From what I read, one should not take Maca a few hours before bedtime, as it can cause insomnia. It's supposed to help your body balance hormone levels through the hypothalamus and pituitary glands. With continued use, it is supposed to promote mental clarity (we all need that!), increase energy levels, and relieve menopausal symptoms such as hot flashes, fatigue, night sweats, mood swings, loss of sexual desire, insomnia, and perimenopausal symptoms. It is also considered a natural alternative to antidepressant medications. (Oh, and it is supposed to help with fertility...but we don't need that one.)

I was having severe sleeping problems, waking up every night around 2:00 or 3:00 a.m., and was unable to fall back to sleep. I also noticed a little depression, anxiety, forgetfulness, and a short attention span during the day. Started taking fish oil capsules and within just a couple of days I was back to my normal self. I know it made the difference because if I forget to take it even one day, my sleep pattern begins to revert back. As long as I'm taking them, I'm sleeping like a log. All the other stuff, anxiety, forgetfulness, etc., is gone as well. All I needed was some good sleep. I would never have dreamed that something so simple could make such a huge difference. They're my little smelly miracle capsules.

I think there's a whole bunch of us on the fish oil bandwagon now! I take a fish/flax blend, though, and I also take the ground flaxseed (two tablespoons) a day. It tastes really good, a whole lot better than the liquid flax oil. I just mix it with a little bit of applesauce and it really tastes good. The flaxseed is another good supplement for menopause.

Has anyone taking the fish oil capsules noticed any change in their bowel movements? It sounds gross, but I have started to notice a little clear mucous with my BMs for the last several days. Could this be from the fish oil? I just started taking them several days ago. I agree that they have helped the anxiety some. I have been trying so many supplements lately, my poor digestive tract probably doesn't know what to do! I have had a little constipation from iron pills, but not too bad. No diarrhea or blood.

I just read the other day that people who get migraines are often magnesium deficient. I found that interesting. I never had a migraine in my life until I hit menopause, and then I started getting the ocular migraines all the time! But after I read about the connection between migraines and magnesium deficiency, it dawned on me that since I've been taking the magnesium, I haven't had one migraine! Oh, I still get a headache once in a while, but think that's work stress.

I am 55 years old and in menopause. I haven't had a period for about three years. About two months ago, I decided to try the natural progesterone cream and rubbed a dab on my forearm each night for about three weeks, then stopped for the last week of the month, as I have read you should do this to mimic your body rhythms. I thought this would help bring my bone density back to a better level and my cholesterol levels. I was having a few hot moments, but not severe, and some interrupted sleeps. These symptoms have disappeared since using the cream. But my question is this: Is it normal for me to be having a full-blown period now? As mentioned above, my last period was about three years ago. I am going to see my doctor, but I'm wondering if anyone else has experienced this and is it normal?

I have heard of that happening when women start to use natural progesterone cream. It can "wake up" some of your hormones. I think it is a good idea that you are checking with your doctor, but I bet the period is from the cream. I started using the cream, thinking it would make my periods lighter, as I was having so much clotting and flooding for days. I really think it made things worse. Each month on the cream, I experienced heavier and longer periods until I had to start the pill to get some control back before I bled to death!

I swear by "live culture" yogurt. Eat one serving (about a cup) of this a day, and it will help diminish intestinal problems (bowel, tummy aches) as well as deter systemic yeast conditions (Candida). As for "natural" menopause treatment, I was on black cohosh for a month, but I found it gave me headaches! I'm trying visualization (mind over matter) to keep hot flashes down, as well as deep breathing and dressing in layers. Of all the menopausal symptoms I detest most, hot flashes are at the top!

I took 5 HTP for a while and I took 100 mg. an hour before bedtime. It did help me to sleep. When I started back on Lexapro, I had to quit taking it, as it can cause seratonin overload if you are taking a SSRI.

I went to my doctor and he put me on Prozac for my depression and mood swings. I was really hoping to find something natural. I take soy for my hot flashes and have for two months, which really helped in that area. Having never suffered from depression, I found it took a toll on me.

🗨 I am a 47 yr old mother of four who is going through perimenopause. I have been for a few years and know exactly what all of you mean! I have had anxiety and heart palpitations. They weren't too bad to begin with, and I handled them with natural progesterone cream, fish oil caps (which have to be natural—do not buy any store brand), Mercury alert (get them in your health food store—Nordic Naturals is a good one!), Mega Foods Maximum Foods vitamins, Heart Response, calcium and magnesium, COQ10, and Vitamin C. I have made a lot of healthy changes in my diet, trying to eat more organic foods. All I drink is either water or organic green tea. I had been feeling pretty good, but all of a sudden I have developed heart flutterings, which are very scary. They come and go, mostly in the afternoon and evening. I am in the middle of my monthly cycle now. Has anyone had this happen in the middle of a cycle? I know it must be hormonal, but why all of a sudden would this happen to me? I have been eating healthier and taking all of my supplements. I have heard of Motherwort helping, and I wonder if anyone tried it yet. I also take Arjuna for my heart and Hawthorne. I have added a mushroom complex with ginger. I have tried anything and everything. Does anything help? I will only deal with this naturally, as I do not go to doctors. Has anyone has tried Motherwort or any other natural products for the heart fluttering? Has anyone tried chasteberry?

🗨 I just had my blood work done and found out I was perimenopausal. I don't want to take any hormone replacement because of all the cancer scares. I have tremors, and I am afraid to take anything that might make them worse. Do you think that taking Maca Root or fish oil will affect the tremors?

🗨 I tried the Maca Root, but I was trying it to boost my libido, which didn't work at all. Someone else I know tried it for the hot flashes, and it didn't help with that either.

🗨 I have been taking Prozac for a little over a week. The doctor said I wouldn't notice any difference for around 28 days. I already notice that I am not as depressed as I was. My sister takes Lexapro and she likes it. I went to a health food store today, the lady there told me to try suma, a mixture of herbs. She said it

75

would help with mood swings and depression. If I could find something to take these extra pounds off I have gained from menopause, I will be happy.

I felt better on the Lexapro right away, even though the doctor told me it would take a week or so to notice any difference. I felt like someone had flipped a switch and I went from darkness to light—it was wonderful! I did stay hungry on the Lexapro, and I switched to Wellbutrin because of that, but with Wellbutrin only, I wasn't depressed but got very angry a lot of the time. After a few months, I added some Lexapro back to it (at night to help me sleep), and the two together are a great combination for me. I have more energy, I don't get nearly as hungry, and I feel better than I do on either of them alone. I have managed to lose a few pounds, so that is good, too! I take a lot of herbs as well, but I have never taken suma. I am not sure what that is for. I will have to look that up.

My doctor changed my hormone pills. Finally last night was the first night I have not had night sweats in a month. Today I have had no hot flashes—a miracle—so the moral of the story is: If your pills aren't working, go back and tell your doctor so he or she can change the type and strength that you are on. I thought I would never feel this way again in my life. What a relief!

I use the Rhodiola Rosasin sometimes, but it is only supposed to help you to deal with stressful situations. It's an adaptegen, so it does a lot of good things in the body as far as helping energy levels, but I don't believe it balances hormones (those are just way too strong to be affected by this herb I believe). But it has helped give me some energy.

I work for a doctor who has known me for 15 years. I told him when all my symptoms seemed to hit the ceiling. He checked me out, as I was afraid I had MS or Parkinson's or a brain tumor. He did blood tests and gave me the once-over. He felt it was menopause and depression most likely caused by the hormone issue. He said to think about Lexapro. He felt it had less side effects but said nothing about the weight gain issue. Then I went to my OB/GYN and asked her about all of this. She didn't want to run hormone tests because she said I was 51 and my hormones were less than they have been in younger years. She said hormone tests sometimes don't show that because at any given time they change. Anyway, she said I have three options: natural alternatives—try a variety of supplements and maybe hit the mark; start HRT to see if it takes the edge off and then we will know if its menopause for sure; or, try Effexor (her anti-depepressant of choice). She thinks the side effects are less than others and you don't get the weight gain like you can from other anti-depressants. I started with the natural options and really did not find it helped a great deal, but I have not been doing it long. I am going to try the HRT to see if I get some relief and, if so, then I know that it's the menopause. Then I can take some time to really research my natural options, as I do not want to take the HRT for any long time frame. You might want to ask your doctor about whether Effexor might be a better option for you if weight gain is something you want to avoid. I just know that at this point in my life it is difficult enough to lose weight and stay healthy.

I went on the Vivelle patch, .0375, along with progesterone cream twice time daily about six months ago. I had numerous (just about debilitating) menopause symptoms. Although they are not gone completely, I feel probably about 80 percent better. I am almost 53 and have had one period (just last month) in the past seven months. I know everyone is different, so I wanted to give you all of my stats!

The ads for Lexapro are so different and unpredictable. They work so differently from each other, and most of them take up to six weeks to reach their full potential. I actually took my mood swings and anxiety a step beyond my regular doctor and gynecologist and started seeing a psych doctor. He prescribed Xanax, which is more of an anti-anxiety medicine. It doesn't take more than about 15 minutes to start working, and you don't take it every day, like the ads indicate. I'm on a low dose, and I only take it when I feel really overwhelmed. You just start feeling like you can handle things. It doesn't make me "high" or anything like that, just more like I'm in control again. You have to be really good about not over-using it, because you can become dependent on it. That was one of my fears when he first prescribed it for me. But it's been almost a year now, and I've had no problems. I also see him about every three weeks. The therapy has really made a huge difference, too. In the beginning, I wasn't sure what I would talk about, but once you get there, it just kind of all falls into place.

I use progesterone cream. I initially started using it to lighten up my periods. After I had my twins and entered my forties, my periods seemed to linger too long. So I started to use it and it helped. I went off it for a while at 43-44 years old and noticed a huge increase in breast tenderness/swelling right before my period and much more painful periods. I would also get night sweats a week before my period. So I went back on the progesterone cream, which helped lessen those PMS-type symptoms. For me, I've found it to be very beneficial.

I have been using progesterone cream for about three months and it does seem to help with the hot flashes and night sweats, it sure doesn't take them away, but I can at least deal with them now. I follow the directions on how much to use. For me, I use an amount between the recommended amount. I would think different brands call for different amounts though. I just did a lot of reading to figure out what one I thought would help most for me.

I tried using progesterone cream because it's the latest "miracle cure" for menopause symptoms. There are several books about how it'll cure everything. I tried it and it didn't help. I have another friend who found that it didn't help her either. The thing to remember is that everyone's hormone balance is different. If you are deficient in progesterone, or all your hormones are high and your estrogen is so high that the progesterone seems way low by comparison, then adding progesterone might help. But if your progesterone is not low, or it is already in balance with your estrogen, then you're just introducing an imbalance by adding a powerful hormone to your body. That is, it might help and it might not. But it isn't "the miracle cure" that every woman needs.

I always hated the time before my period when my progesterone was at its highest. Major PMS symptoms! Then when I started HRT, I found that the estrogen part of the cycle really helped, but when I used the progesterone pills every month as required to induce a period, I felt like I was back in PMS mode again. Now that I am definitely past menopause, my doctor is letting me use progesterone every six months to induce a period. This is much better. He keeps telling me that if I agree to a hysterectomy, I won't have to take the progesterone at all, but I am not going for that drastic a measure unless it's absolutely medically necessary.

I use progesterone oil. The cream just didn't work for me. The oil absorbs much better. Anyway, I get incredible relief from progesterone oil. I did an at-home saliva test that I purchased at a pharmacy and had the results mailed to me. My estrogen was higher than my progesterone at the time in my cycle that they should both be around the same amount. I always believed I was estrogen dominant because of my symptoms. It took about two to three months of use to get the full benefit, but it has made all the difference for me. I use it around day 12 of my cycle until the start of my period, and then I stop. My depression is gone, my tender/sore breasts are gone, my lack of energy is gone. In addition to the progesterone oil, I also added a high potency magnesium, a high potency vitamin D3, and a very good probiotic. I eliminated caffeine from my diet. No more coffee, tea, chocolate. I feel so much better than I have in a long time. I was miserable for over a year. I had horrible GERD, slept constantly, was moody and grumpy. I couldn't concentrate, felt foggy headed, and had terrible anxiety. I think I finally found the right combo for me.

I started HRT about a month ago. I was having hot flashes one after the next and felt like I had a constant fever, was nauseated, and had night sweats with waking up at all times of the night, which made me irritable. I am on Premarin (estrogen only), and we started out at .3, which is a small dosage. I am now at .625, and we have decided to stick with this since it is working. I have noticed the weight gain (I can use the extra breast weight). I enrolled in the YMCA and, now that I am feeling much better, I plan on getting into a regular exercise program and drink lots of fluids like water. I think you and your doctor just have to try the different strengths until you can find the right one. I asked my doctor if the hormone test can determine the strength I need, and he told me two women can have the same estrogen level but one can have hot flashes while the other has none. To each her own, but I feel much better and can finally function again so I am going to stick with this and perhaps, in time, try to lower the dosage.

I am almost 53, and through my late forties I used the progesterone cream (over the counter) and felt totally fine. I had no other symptoms but felt like a radiator. After all, I thought that was what menopause was all about—hot flashes—even though I had started to read about it to get "prepared." I pretty much thought that everything I was reading about was to get rid of that and maybe a few other minor symptoms. Anyway, when I was 50, it hit me one day like a lead balloon and I have felt unwell ever since in varying degrees. I have many of those 35 symptoms of menopause, if you've ever heard about those. I could never have been prepared to feel so different and unhealthy, and I have been checked for many other things, as I was not convinced this was menopause--it's such a well-kept secret in my opinion! As for the saliva test, I had one ordered and read by a doctor on two occasions. The reason your doctor may not have shed much light on your test results is that the doctor may just not be versed on it. Even the doctor I am seeing for bioidentical hormones prefers blood work and is not versed on the saliva test. Dr. Christine Nothrup, one of the leading menopause doctors—you may have seen her on TV and she has written numerous books—no longer feels the same way about the saliva tests as she once did.

I have been on Amberen for almost four months. I feel great. I never really had the hot flashes at night, so I can't say they relieved them. I do sleep better about 90 percent of the time. I really am no longer depressed, and my anxiety has subsided except for little ones once in a while, but nothing to annoy me. I also take a multi/mineral/herb supplement along with fish/flax/borage and have been feeling great. It is not HRT. I will finish my 90-day supply and then wait three months and go back on for another 90 days. They explained it to me why they suggest this, but I cannot put it in my own words. I will see how I feel once I finish the 90 days. I may need to stay on it longer!

I always was a worrier, but I wouldn't call myself really having full-blown anxiety until I hit perimenopause. All of a sudden, I had panic attacks while driving on the freeway, and I just couldn't do it anymore. I also felt like I was coming unglued at times, when I hadn't ever really felt like that before or to that extent. But when I starting going through menopause, I was so sad and depressed, and I had a hopeless feeling, not to mention the anxiety, not being able to sleep, the morning fatigue, you name it! I went to my gynecologist and told him that I threw in the towel, I needed help or I was going off the deep end. I never wanted to be on hormones, so he suggested that I try Lexapro. It made a different person out of me in literally a couple of days! It cured everything for me, from anxiety, depression, hot flashes, night sweats, you name it. Not everyone can take antidepressants, but I was one of the lucky ones who could. I am still taking it and haven't had a period in about three years, but I am afraid of not taking it!

I take an all-in-one menopause supplement and it contains (amongst nine other vitamins and minerals) 60 mg. magnesium, which, according to the box, gives me 20 percent of the RDA here in England. It also gives me 158 mg. of calcium, which is more than the recommended 2:1 ratio of calcium to magnesium. The only other supplement I take is an omega 3 bomb. I like to think I get whatever else I need from my diet, which I believe is pretty healthy.

I am working with a compound pharmacist. She recommended 400-500 mg. of chelated magnesium. Since I have been taking the chelated magnesium vs. the regular, I no longer have very loose stools (sorry to be gross, but magnesium helps with constipation, but the regular kind does the opposite). She also told me to take it three hours before bedtime. It is supposed to help with sleep, but it hasn't with me. I sleep sometimes and wake up frequently and go right back to sleep, and other times I am up for hours—no rhyme or reason to any of it!

I've been doing some reading and was surprised to find that magnesium oxide (which is the most common magnesium in supplements) is poorly absorbed. Only about 4 percent of the elemental magnesium is absorbed. Magnesium citrate and magnesium gluconate seem to be the best absorbed. Magnesium citrate will cause loose stools. The magnesium gluconate, apparently doesn't cause as much issues with loose stools. I am going to try a powder form called Natural Calm. From what I've read, it has the best absorption percentage.

I am on the Vivelle patch. I am also on progesterone cream, which I was told is imperative to use while using the patch (not necessarily the cream, but I was told we need the estrogen/progesterone combination). I was also told I might be worse before better and I found that to be true. They didn't want to make any adjustments until I had been on it a full three months. The nausea in the middle of the night was terrible and would last hours. That was attributed to the progesterone cream which was then cut in half, and now the nausea is gone. I have been on the bio-identical hormones for six months. I was on the regular hormones for six months prior to that. My assessment for myself is: I was about 50 percent better on the regular hormones; I am about 60-75 percent better on the bio-identical hormones; and I just feel all around better using hormones that have been prescribed specifically for me as a result of my blood work and being monitored on a quarterly basis and using plant derived hormones. Wish I didn't have to use them at all, but the quality of my life was greatly affected-short of going into all of the gory details!

I started Amberen after much research (as much as I could find). I seem to be doing better since being on it. My headaches are disappearing, I am sleeping better, and overall I just feel a little better, calmer, focused. My anxiety/depression has diminished somewhat even when it is gloomy out, which was always a factor for me I think. At least I know I am guaranteed my money back if not satisfied. I don't want to really speculate just yet on how I actually feel, as it is only my fourth day (and this could just be a few good days I have had) and I want to wait at least one to two weeks before seeing any real results. I also read that a bunch of vitamins and minerals, Balanced Formula One, is supposed to be good. Look into it if you are not sure about Amberen.

Q I am 55 and have been taking Amberen for a full three weeks. I am at the start of my fourth week. I was hesitant to take Amberen because it is so new, but I wanted relief bad and nothing else worked for me. Amberen is quick to work. In the first two days of taking Amberen, my hot flashes and night sweats seemed to worsen, but after three days they were pretty much gone. In the first week, my brain fog was gone and the fatigue with it. I am no longer dead tired when I get home from work. Amberen has made a huge difference in the way I was feeling before. I was feeling so awful every day and it showed. My energy level was so low that it was a great struggle just to cook, clean, work, or do anything else for that matter. Now I can do all of those things with energy to spare. It hasn't improved on my sleep yet. I still get only about three to four hours of sleep, but the quality of sleep is much better. Maybe that part will take a little longer. I no longer have vaginal dryness either. There's a slight change in libido. So far there are no negatives.

Q I'm still taking my bio-estrogen cream. I tried the patches before, and they made me so sick, even in the smallest dose. I can't seem to tolerate anything anymore or even the vitamins, supplements, and medications I used to take. It's like my body is reacting to everything. I, too, get the palpitations and sometimes I get anxiety really bad. I'm not sure if it's the estrogen in general. My doctor measures my levels by blood tests, and I just had my hormones checked by saliva. I know I'm low on estrogen. It feels like I have no fluid in my entire body! I'm considering trying that supplement called Amberen instead.

Q I went on low-dosage HRT for several years when it became apparent that I was starting perimenopause. During this time, I had no problems with the usual symptoms that people here report. Then one month it felt as though I was taking a placebo when I experienced the same hot flashes and unsettled moods that I had experienced before I started taking HRT. Then I realized that the problem wasn't that the pills were placebos, but that they plus my own hormone production didn't amount to enough in total. I went back to my doctor and got a stronger prescription.

I felt extremely unwell over the past two years with all of the symptoms described. After visiting numerous doctors to rule out everything else, I first went on regular HRT and, in September, bioidentical HRT. I have had both blood tests and saliva tests. Part of what determined the course of action was that I was still getting my period sporadically. I will be retested next week and, depending on what I tell them my symptoms are now coupled with the test results and in addition I have not had a period since starting the bioidentical hormones in September, this will determine is any change is needed to the prescribed HRT. I am using Vivelle and an estrogen patch and progesterone cream. I am feeling about 75 percent better, thank goodness. I have had some bad days, which, I am guessing, are due to my own body's fluctuation because it still seems almost cyclical.

I myself have been going through menopause for almost eight years, and water retention has been one of many of the symptoms from menopause that has affected me. My doctor prescribed water tablets. They help a bit, but I'm still bloated, more so in my legs, which I agree can cause pain.

I'm almost ten years into menopause. When in early menopause, I suffered with many yeast infections and UTIs. A female physician suggested eating yogurt with "live active cultures" every day. You can find the live culture info on the container. It's in small print, and you do have to look for it. My yeast infections cleared up quickly and also the UTIs have not come back. Today, if I do not eat yogurt daily, then I chew an acidophilus tablet. I purchase the tablets at any drug store and they are not expensive. When I started into menopause, I tried to go with the natural alternative route. But, with way too many intense hot flashes, dry with vaginal atrophy, bladder leakage, tiredness, no sleep, inability to think straight, and starting to age fast, I gave in to HRT. I have never regretted it. I waited four years and wish I had made my decision earlier. Over six years ago, I started HRT and PremPro. My female OB/GYN also started me on a direct application of Premarin cream. The Premarin cream did help with the dryness greatly, but I also contributed it to staying on the HRT. And today if I experience some dryness, then I use the cream for two to three days. It might be months between applications. I have not had a UTI in six years, either. However, it is painful to try to have sex. It appears my tissues are very thin. My husband and I do have a great relationship because there are alternate ways to be physically close.

⬤ I take vitamin D3 (4,000 IU daily) and really think it's helping, but I had a deficiency in the first place. One thing I've noticed is that I'm not getting my annual bout of depression this year. It usually hits somewhere around September or October, and it hasn't shown up yet. I attribute that to the vitamin D. It's also helped a lot with my joint pain. If you're having tingling, it might be a good idea to have your B levels tested. One of the signs of low B12 is tingling in the hands and/or feet. It might also explain the nerve pain. Regardless of what the range is on the test, the optimal level for health should be up around 1,000. If your level is lower than that, you should start taking sublingual B12 lozenges. Don't worry about taking too much. Your body will just eliminate what it doesn't need.

⬤ I have tried many multi vitamins, and the worst of it for me was swallowing the dang things and then trying to digest the huge pill with all the stomach problems I've had since becoming perimenopausal. The one that I have finally found that is easy to digest is Viactiv. It's a multi vitamin made for women by women. And the vitamins come in soft, chocolate flavored chews. Now mind you, they do not taste as yummy as a Dove chocolate, but they are much easier for me to tolerate than the hard, gigantic vitamins offered by other companies. I also take an Ester C, 250 mg. Magnesium, and a 1,000 mg. fish oil capsule daily. When I remember, I take calcium at night, also in a chewable by Viactiv. These seem to work for me so far!

⬤ I first took estrogen and it was bio-identical in 1998, one year after my periods stopped. The only symptoms I had then were hot flashes. I was also battling systemic yeast which I had had for 18 or more years and was on and off Diflucan for ten years, so some of my other symptoms like gas, some muscle aches now and then, sort of overlapped my menopausal symptoms, but I was starting to have painful sex. My doctor put me on bio-identical HRT. At first my hot flashes increased, my painful sex got better, and my overall feelings got worse. I was tired, achy, goofy-headed, slow, and still didn't feel good. I stopped taking them. In 2000 I tried Pregnelone and felt better on that but it made my heart pound and race, and I couldn't handle that so I stopped. My painful sex got worse and other symptoms showed up, fight-or-flight feelings, the tops of my legs hurt to go up stairs, more flashes, but HRT only made it worse, so I learned to live with myself and ignored the problems and went on with my life, which wasn't bad. I had a lot of energy, that never changed. I was always happy and constantly on the go. Then in early 2003 I felt tired all the time, sex was nonexistent, too painful, and panic attacks were more frequent. My doctor put me back on bioidenticals and that time they worked. I felt great for three weeks, no panic attacks, no muscle problems, sex was better, then all of a sudden my heart screwed up. It was awful, hard beats, irregular, racing, and I thought I was having a heart attack. I was at ER twice and had many tests for one year. They said I was nuts! I was afraid to go anywhere and, when I did, I would be so scared and nervous, something I had no control over even when I tried. I blamed it on the hormones, but it may have been going to happen anyway. So, I stopped the HRT. My heart has improved since then, but I have tons of other terrible menopause symptoms, thus my posts. It's awful, isn't it? I want my life back so badly. I want to try the HRT again but am scared to death it will screw up my heart again, and that is worse for me than all the symptoms. Well, the nerve pain is just as bad, when half the time my body feels like there is nothing below my neck, not numb, just heavy and not there. My legs hurt so much I can hardly walk, and I have constant stomach and abdomen pain.

I take calcium 1,000 mg, magnesium 500 mg. with vitamin.D. That helps the heart palpitations and works like a mild tranquilizer to relax nerves. Also, I take standardized black cohosh 40 mg. for the sweats (must say Standardized and be 40 mg, not the others), Centrum Silver multi-vitamin, flax seed oil caps (or sometimes salmon oil caps for the Omegas), and cinnamon caps to keep sugars level. These things seem to help, especially the calcium and magnesium. The dose for 1,000 mg., which is four caps a day, so I carry them with me and take one about 10:00 a.m., another about 3:00 in the afternoon (or whenever I get nervous or jittery feelings in the afternoon), and then two before bedtime to help me sleep. Since I am now three years postmenopause, I take the black cohosh at night because that is really the time that I will get a flash or two if I get one at all, which always seems to be while sleeping. This was all from reading about all of this that I decided this was the formula for me. My doctor says it's all okay with her, though she has never understood why I want to just go natural and put up with some of the things like the mood swings rather than take an anti-depressant. I have had so many friends and relatives go on them and have worse problems develop that I just thought that part out and hope it goes away.

🗨 I am three years postmenopausal and still get the racing heart palpitations. The fix for me was taking calcium/magnesium in a 2:1 ratio. I take 1,000 mg. calcium with 500 mg. Magnesium, and vitamin D, all in capsule form (the dose is six a day, so I take three at night so the palpitations and jittery feelings don't bother me and the other three during the day any time I choose, especially if I get any palpitations during the day that remind me). This has definitely saved me a lot of anxiety. I went to the ER when the palpitations and jittery feelings first started. They ran an EKG, which was normal and has remained normal. I just had this year's physical a couple days ago, and my EKG was the same as usual. They say that the racing palpitations are caused by a shortage of magnesium. Because I need the calcium and vitamin D anyway, I buy the caps that have them all together. Just remember the 2:1 ratio with the calcium/magnesium.

🗨 I've been going around and around this for some time and still haven't been able to get myself to take the doctor recommended antidepressant, Lexapro. I am taking HRT. It became such a quality of life issue; I felt I had to do something about the hot flashes, sleeplessness, low libido, etc. I have not had depression in my life, but am really now struggling since last summer. I keep hoping that with diet and exercise I will not have to take antidepressants, but here I am again in tears for no apparent reason and additional hot flashes as well. I'm starting to regret not listening to my doctor and am sitting on the fence about this for all the obvious reasons not to take antidepressants.

🗨 I took black cohosh for night sweats for four years. but it has to say on the label "Black Cohosh 40 mg. Standardized." If it doesn't say standardized or if it is different mgs., it is the wrong stuff and won't work (it has to do with the part of the plant and the controlled dosage). I stopped taking it once to see if they had gone away naturally, and they came back within 48 hours. I went back to the cohosh and they went away again. They were not always gone but were at least mild (meaning if I had some, they lasted a matter of a minute or two). Also, I take 1,000 mg. calcium with 500 mg. magnesium with vitamin D which is total in six capsules. I take one in the morning, two in the afternoon, and three at bedtime along with Centrum Silver since I am postmenopausal.

I have been using an estrogen patch for several years. I am past menopause, so I take progesterone only every six months. The estrogen patch has been much easier to use than the pills I used to take. The only problem I have had is with the first kind that I tried. I became allergic to the glue of the patch. My doctor switched me to a different brand and I have had no problems with this one. I feel much better with estrogen. My moods are calmer, I have very few hot flashes, and my joints seem to have less stiffness.

I have been on Lexapro for five years. My hysterectomy led directly to menopause. The drug is great with no side effects for me (everyone is different). I had been on other antidepressants before, but all of them had severe side effects. Warning: Talk to your doctor before stopping as you do need to wean off!

Vaginal dryness is when your vagina is no longer naturally producing the mucus that allows for easy and pleasurable intercourse. When my hormones got too low, intercourse felt like my vagina was being scoured with sandpaper. KY-Jelly doesn't help. Some women may have an easier transition than others. I use a vaginal cream that has estrogen in it. Ask your gynecologist about this. It can be used by people who cannot take estrogen pills or patches because of their risk factors (family history of heart problems or breast cancer, etc.). The estrogen in the vaginal cream stays local and doesn't affect the rest of the body. It works wonders. I have also seen someone post that they use olive oil in the vagina.

I'm 35 and will soon have a hysterectomy for endometriosis and a fibroid tumor of the uterus. My gynecologist gave me a shot of Lupron a month ago to be sure that the pain I've been having is in fact endometriosis. Both ovaries have to be removed to end the possibility of that problem returning. The decision also relates to my history of cancer (breast cancer in 2004). I'm finally experiencing symptoms of menopause, caused by the Lupron, and will probably experience such symptoms after my surgery. I've begun getting hot flashes.

I have had counseling and medications for 16 years, due to obsessive- compulsive disorder and anxiety. I was uncertain about taking drugs at first, then the doctor explained to me that I felt the way I did because I was missing the chemical it took to regulate my body. I needed to add it to feel normal again. To not add the chemical I needed was the same as withholding insulin from a diabetic. I was at the point where everything was regulated, and I only saw a therapist every six months to reassure him and myself that all was well. Perimenopause came around and undid everything, so back to the therapist I went. It helps that he's known me for years and knows what is normal behavior and what is not. I take Effexor and supplement with Xanax as needed. I have taken Xanax as needed for 16 years and was at the point where as needed meant hardly ever! Now as needed means daily, and I'm not crazy about that, but I am still at the same low dose I was prescribed 16 years ago. I tried bio-identical hormones, but they did not work for me. They made me more anxious and depressed. I guess the point I'm trying to make is medication can work, especially used in conjunction with counseling. I wouldn't go to a doctor that prescribed a drug and then just wrote me off.

I was on a low dosage of HRT for years when I was in perimenopause. Then one day it felt like someone had made a mistake at the pharmacy by giving me placebos. It felt like I wasn't taking any hormones at all and my symptoms came back with a vengeance. After I calmed down (one of the symptoms of low hormones is, of course, freaking out abut everything), I went back to the doctor and had my dosage upped. Much better. Another thing you might try for depression is Vitamin D3. I'm reading more and more about how people in the Western world are very deficient in it. Most of us don't get much sunlight because we're indoors all day. And I live in northern Germany where the sun don't shine but seldom! I was suffering from seasonal affective disorder (SAD) every winter when I lived in California, and when we moved here I started getting depression earlier and earlier every year until one year it didn't lift at all. Since I have been taking Vitamin D3, I have no more depression. I'm still fundamentally a cynic and pessimist at heart, but now I can actually see the bright side of things more often than not.

I had a total hysterectomy two years ago this October. I was finally put on HRT because I couldn't stand the results of being in full-blown menopause. I am on the Vivelle patch (v-dot) and love it. My hair has thinned significantly, but my hair was always pin straight and a little thin to begin with. When my hair is completely wet when washing it, I notice there's not much hair thickness-wise and it freaks me out. It does fall out more if you dye it, too, only the day you first dye it. My hair is beginning to grow longer now, and I noticed it wasn't' growing as quickly as it used to. There are so many physical changes in menopause, even being on hormones. I can't imagine what would happen to my body if I weren't on the hormone patch.

A friend suggested I replace milk with soy, as this is protein rather than dairy, and it's recommended to help alleviate hot flushes. Well, I have to say, so far so good. I can't drink it on its own, but a bit heated up for a cup of coffee seems to be doing the trick. I've also replaced my dairy yogurts with soy ones, and the hot flushes seem to have subsided. Let's hope it's not just coincidence

When I was going through perimenopause, I started getting bad migraine headaches around the time I should have a period. I never had migraines until then. Many women I worked with all complained of their migraines and, of course me never having one, always thought "take a couple Advil and settle down" until I started getting them. Sometimes they would last two or three days. They turned out to be hormonal migraines. I went to my doctor and got on HRT low-dose and haven't had one migraine headache since. There is a connection. Talk to your GP about it for some relief.

Q When I had a hysterectomy two years ago, they took everything but one ovary, probably hoping I would not go into menopause as soon as possible. I did very slowly. It started with the hot flashes, really bad ones. My doctor put me on a low dose of Provera and Premarin. They help a little bit. But my hair is dry, falling out more, and I have vaginal dryness, severe migraines, breast enlargement, sleeplessness, weight gain, swings, and anxiety. What my concern is the migraines. I have had them since I was four years old, and I am now 46. Over the last year they have gotten worse. I am now waking up with a severe migraine almost daily, and Zomig or Maxalt helps. I also take Tylenol 3 on occasion. Even when I am at work I will get a migraine. I work at a physiotherapy office. I am getting very desperate. Migraines are interfering with my job.

Q I took Ativan for about three months. It did work to control the anxiety, but my biggest problem was that it left me so tired. I also had real worries about being on it too long and becoming reliant. I slowly weaned myself off it and went to natural remedies. I would say that short term, it's great for helping control the anxiety while you search for what else will work for you. It frees up your mind so that you're not crippled by the anxiety while you're trying to figure out what to try next. I wouldn't be comfortable long term with it, but then I'm pretty anti-drug.

Q My doctor put me back on HRT—3 mg. Premarin. I stopped taking my 6.25 Premarin three years ago after being on it for 14 years. (At the age of 41, my ovaries were removed and my uterus had been removed when I was 26). My estrogen level was 7 on the blood test, and my doctor said that women who have had the same surgeries usually test out at 27. He said that my levels were very low. Because I am experiencing some vaginal dryness, etc., he thought that this might be a good idea. My husband says since I stopped taking the Premarin three years ago, I have basically fallen apart. I had lots of problems, like aches, pains, dryness, and so forth. To start taking hormones again is a hard decision for me. I am afraid of the possible side effects. That is why I stopped taking them after 14 years of being on them.

● I'm 48 and started Provera this month. I'm taking it because my periods kept getting closer together. I'm to take it on day 12 of my cycle for 12 days. I'm not having any issues on it yet, but I've only taken it for six days total. I got my period on day 13 last month, so I'm past that this month. I guess the I should get it a few days after I stop, and a that will be day 27 or so. I recall that my gynecologist said to give it a try, but it may not work. So I'm thinking this means that I may still experience short cycles even while on it. I think that maybe our hormones are going to do what they please, and I've also read that Provera can cause menstrual irregularities, which makes no sense if they're giving it to us, so we become more regular. My gynecologist also said that over the past year, I have a progesterone deficiency, so I guess taking Provera should help me.

● I've been on Femhart for about four years and love it! I have no problems at all. There are two versions of it, one of which is a low dose. I'm on the regular one. When I first switched to it from birth control pills, my gynecologist told me I would probably have some bleeding around period time for the next two to three months. That never happened. I never had another period! It has been wonderful! I recommend it highly. I started my periods at age 10 and went on Femhart at age 56. It was darned well time to quit having periods!

● I take Buspar. It has helped tremendously. Three years ago I got hit with anxiety big time. I couldn't eat or sleep and was put on a couple of antidepressants, but side effects were too bad. I was put on Buspar, and it worked wonders. However, last year when the anxiety came back, I was put on a higher dose and it seemed to work well. This is the time of year that it hits the worse. I did have some breakthrough anxiety in December, about 10 days before my last period. I have only had two periods in the last 11 months. Also, I seem to be dealing with some depression now. This is not fun.

I use a bioidentical progesterone cream and found it did take time for it to become totally effective. My container says that some women see results in two weeks, while others can take up to two months to really see results. I started seeing great changes after two months. I now feel totally fine, all my issues are pretty well gone.

Inderal for me has worked wonders for migraine and high blood pressure. I have been taking it for 18 years. The difference in the way my doctor wants me to take the tablets is 20 mg. four times daily. That way Inderal levels stay consistent throughout the day. If you still get breakthrough migraines, you may want to tell your doctor you want to switch over to four times daily, as it works great for me. Inderal is also prescribed for some women to relieve hot flashes.

I am on fish oil and multi vitamins. I also take 400 mg. of B2 for migraines. (My neurologist told me to try this.) I don't get the really bad migraines, but I do get the neck pain every month. I have taken Motrin for it, but it doesn't seem to do anything. I guess it's hormone related.

I am 42 and am in full-blown menopause. I started HRT a year ago. I do not like to take chemicals, so I was taking half of each pill (I forgot their names—estrogen and progesterone?). Well, I have HPV and am worried about the cc thing. I started taking some natural supplements and quit the HRT cold turkey this past Saturday. Yesterday I started getting crampy and a little bit of what looked like old blood was on the tissue when I wiped. Today I am a little crampy but no blood. This morning I woke up with a fuzzy head and have felt awful all morning. I finally gave in and took two of the halves of HRT. Is this normal stuff for withdrawals? I am freaking out. I am seeing my doctor on Monday for my yearly, but I think the anxiety will do me in before than.

About two years ago I sought a gynecologist that deals with bioidentical hormones . We tested my hormone levels with a saliva test that I purchased from her office. You do the test at home and mail it to the lab. They send the results to the doctor who will then write a prescription depending on your hormone levels or lack thereof (mine were all deficient). The cost varies depending on how many hormones you are testing. The first one I did included estrogen, progesterone, testosterone, DHEA, and cortisol. I think it was $150-$200. Yes, it's expensive. I think my insurance covered part of it, but not all. And I have yet to get them to accept to pay for my compounded hormones. Anyway, if you don't have a doctor that will do this, and if you can find a compounding pharmacy, you might inquire if the pharmacist can read the results of your test for you and recommend the prescription, which you can then get through your doctor. (You can buy the saliva tests online, just do a search.) My pharmacy actually mails my hormones to me (I'm still using the same one from before I moved.) I don't know if that can be done to the UK, but you'd still need to get the testing done. It makes it easier if you can find a gynecologist in the first place that is on board with all of this. We have to be our own advocates because there aren't any drug companies out there that can make a buck off us poor menopausal women except with the nasty HRT that is currently on the market.

Technically, going off HRT doesn't actually postpone menopause, because HRT doesn't do anything to restore your ability to make eggs. What HRT does do is postpone the symptoms of menopause. You're still in menopause even while you're taking the hormones. You're just treating the symptoms. I'm 57 (oops, I just realized that I'll be 58 in less than two weeks) and I've been on some form of HRT since my early forties. I started obvious menopause symptoms (hot flashes, no periods for a few months, drying skin, etc.) when I was 39. So I've been using substitute hormones for over 15 years. I've discussed this with my doctor, who says that, theoretically, women with no risk factors (history of cancer or heart problems or other things) can stay on HRT for years. The important thing if you continue the HRT is to have regular doctor visits to make sure that your body is doing okay on the hormones. And you might consider using the lowest dosage you can tolerate to keep the symptoms at bay. If you really want to stop the hormones, then tapering slowly over several months is a must. If and when you decide to stop HRT, your body has to adjust to living without the hormones. In that sense, it's as if you had postponed menopause.

I went off birth control pills in October and my skin looks bad. It was never great to start with, but I know what you mean by your skin looking older. I have read that when we start to lose estrogen, we lose collagen in our skin, too. Being off the pill, the estrogen levels will decrease. I am sure once you are on HRT for a while, your skin appearance will probably improve because you will have some estrogen back in your system again. I have acne as well, and the pill helped some, but now it's back in full force. It's the pits to look bad and feel bad, too!

Palpitations are often part of menopause, but it is also sometimes caused by things we take from over-the-counter to self-medicate some menopausal symptoms that seem unlikely, such as Motrin. With menopause come severe headaches and joint and muscle pain, though we don't often equate those pains consciously with menopause. We simply use what we have in the medicine cabinet. Frequently the implied dosage is two every six to eight hours. But we also know that when we've had, for example, dental work, the doctor has prescribed prescription dosages that appear to equate to four of the non-prescription. Non-prescription Motrin in large doses (not just Motrin, but also Tylenol and their generic equivalents) are not the same chemical structure as those via prescription. Over time these do some pretty dangerous stuff to the human body: Severe palpitations, breathlessness, difficulty urinating (slow stream and a feeling the bladder still holds urine)—these are some of the ones we become conscious of, but there are other more silent problems, too. One of the scariest aspects of menopause is that doctors have a hard time treating symptoms and that affects the sufferer to find ways to self-medicate. Take a look at any medications you are presently taking. If you can eliminate any other offenders, then the symptoms are probably menopausal, but I would recommend talking to your doctor regardless!

I'm 50 now and did get off the pill back in September. I was afraid that my hot flashes and other menopause symptoms would worsen. I began taking Enjuvia, conjugated estrogens. I feel fantastic! While I was on the pill, it was as though I had no moisture in my body. My vagina, my complexion, and my skin were dry and dull. My sex drive was completely gone. But since taking estrogens, my periods have been extremely light and come every 40 to 60 days. They last two or three days. My sex drive is back and no longer uncomfortable. My skin is baby soft and (don't laugh) my breasts have gotten perkier, and my nipples are soft, whereas on the pill they were dry and scaly. Yuck! For once in many years, I feel like a real woman. I even feel sexy. Oh, and I've lost ten pounds, simply by substituting a big dinner with a snack instead. That could be ice cream, popcorn, or cereal, anything you love, as long as it is not a heavy meal. I couldn't lose an ounce while on the pill.

Q My trip through perimenopause has so far been crazy. I have over time gained some great habits that do help me out, like cheap, inexpensive ways to pamper myself because I want to, need to, and deserve to. Please don't read any of these things I do and say, "I can't because..." The more you say it, the more your brain believes it. To some, this may sound silly, but for others it may really be just what the doctor should have ordered: powdered milk bath (even if its 2:00 a.m., we're not sleeping anyway) for about $1.99; candles/votives (ten for $1) in the bath room; soft music (I have gained a whole new respect for classical music); foot/heel scrubber (I got for 99 cents) which just makes my feet feel better; cranberry juice drink from a cheap wine glass—I'm telling you, its good for the soul; lavender body spray (I bought at the dollar store and spray my pillows at night); Dove soap (the blue kind. "calming night")—just the scent of it is worth it; child's ball (I purchased from the grocery store, not an expensive exercise ball)—I put the ball between my knees and squeeze while I am at the computer—it's exercise! (I also sometimes just hold it out in my hands and squeeze it to relieve tension); word scrambles or puzzles get my mind focused, a brain exercise; and small flat rocks (I got from the riverbed) which I put into warm water (not boiling) and let them warm, then take them out, lie down, and place the rocks on my tummy where it cramps, and/or on my neck and legs and arms (who needs $50-an-hour spa?). A friend of mine said her mom makes the rocks cold and uses them during a hot flash. These are just a few. I don't do these every day, but I think the important thing is taking time for yourself. We all go through so much, even what's considered mild is still a major blow from feeling normal.

● I'm at the stage where I get a period one month but then go two months without. I use the progesterone cream on days 14-26 of my cycle when I get my period. On the months where I don't get a period, I use it starting on the first of the month and then stop for five days at the end of the month. This last month, I did get a period, so I'm going to use it when I hit day 14, stop at day 26, and assume I'm getting a period. If I don't get one, then I'll restart the cream as close as possible to the first of the month. I have to admit that I do find it a bit of a juggling act now with periods all over the place.

● I can tell you what quantity I'm taking right now. I don't think the brand particularly matters, although you should make sure that the coating on your oil base vitamins doesn't contain di-alpha tachoceryaphyl acetate. I'm using mostly the Jamieson brand vitamins. I currently take: two times daily, Omega 3-6-9 Biocomplex which contains 400 mg. each of flax oil, borage oil, and fish oil; just before bedtime, 250 mg. tablet of magnesium, one multi-vitamin, and 400 UI vitamin E; one time a day, 1,000 mg. Evening Primrose oil and 1,000 mg. Mega B complex. I also use Natural Progesterone cream on days 14-26 of my cycle. Slo-mag would likely be the slow release form of magnesium. You can get most vitamins these days in a slow release format.

● Vaginal dryness is a naturally-occurring condition experienced by women of many ages. Its symptoms may include not just dryness, but itching, burning, soreness and irritation (called vaginitis), as well as discomfort during and after sex. When the vaginal lining becomes thinner, there is a decrease in natural lubrication during arousal. The most common cause of feminine dryness is a depletion of estrogen that occurs as women enter midlife and move toward menopause, or after a hysterectomy. Other causes may include infection, loss of estrogen after childbirth, side effects of medications, immune disorders, surgery, and chemotherapy or radiation treatment. Bacterial and/or yeast infections can often temporarily set off a chemical imbalance that causes vaginal dryness and irritation (vaginitis), as can douching. For some menopausal or premenopausal women, doctors will prescribe estrogen therapy, which may be provided externally through patches, creams, other topical delivery systems, or internally through pills. For women who are not receiving estrogen therapy for relief from menopausal symptoms or who simply want a more natural alternative, the most frequently used method of self-care is a vaginal lubricant and/or feminine moisturizer. There is a new one called Soft Touch.

When I first started taking Evening Primrose (when my cycles were gushers), I took one capsule a day, 1,000 mg. each. Within two to three days they slowed down. I take it all month long and have not had a heavy period since, for approximately one year. I now take three a week, all month, at the suggestion of a naturopathic doctor. I am assuming because they are oil based it stays in your body fat longer than something that is water soluble. I never had one side effect, and I have trouble with everything.

I've been going through symptoms for five years. My periods stopped two years ago. But hot flashes, anxiety, and general crappy feeling got bad this fall (I am 51). I saw my gynecologist in January, and he suggested HRT (PremPro) lowest dose. I decided to try it, took one pill every other day (I wanted to see if just a little would help). In a week I felt great emotionally, no hot flashes, etc., but by two weeks I had put on a couple pounds, had low back pain, my ovaries hurt, and I had a yeast infection. I stopped taking them. I really wish I would not have to choose feeling okay emotionally and having physical problems or deciding which symptoms I can best tolerate. I do not want to battle the weight issue. I took birth control pills in my mid-twenties and I always carried five to ten extra pounds with them; when I stopped taking them, the weight returned.

I was put on HRT once and within days had a horrible period and legs cramps. My doctor told me to stop it immediately, and months later we tried a different patch. The same thing happened. I had a period within days that lasted over a month and horrific leg cramps. I was already through menopause for almost two years and went on it for the night sweats. After this, I opted to go it alone. I am now three years into menopause and have no symptoms, but boy was it difficult for the first two-and-a-half years.

I was on birth control pills for nine months to control my heavy, non-stop periods. It worked great. I stopped the pill last fall and have had two periods since October. One was fairly light, and my last one was heavy for several days but stopped on its own. I am 52 and really didn't feel comfortable taking the pill for any longer. I hope the time I was on the pill helped to regulate my periods, and maybe now they will just slowly go away!

I've been using compounded hormones for about nine months and still have times when symptoms seem to reappear or when I just feel simply blah. Then there are those times when I feel almost 100 percent normal again, such as for about two weeks back in the spring. Recently I received the results from my saliva test and my progesterone, estrogen, testosterone, and DHEA are below the minimum range. Since I've been taking progesterone for months and my levels are still below the range, there is now the question as to why my body isn't absorbing the hormones. I think that this hormone business is strictly guess work, it's not a science, and it will require monitoring and tweaking. Although my doctor is basing treatment upon my symptoms and saliva test result, there are doctors who disagree with the validity of the saliva test. Yes, this is all guess work, but I'm thankful that we do have options because no treatment is not an option for many of us.

I was on Effexor for two years and recently went off of it primarily because I wanted to try life without it. I, too, have a huge problem with anxiety. I liked Effexor, but the withdrawal was pure hell and I gained weight. I'm thinking of trying Cymbalta because I'm also being plagued with lots of aches and pains and have been diagnosed with fibromyalgia. It's gotten much worse since going off the antidepressants and entering menopause. I'm almost 55 and my last period was in October. I'm also on a compounded estrogen/progesterone/testosterone cream. But I really haven't seen much difference. I've never had hot flashes (well I think I've had two actually), but the anxiety is killing me.

● I was on Effexor, 75 mg., for two years. I found it actually produced night sweats for me. I am 54 and had never had night sweats until I went on the Effexor.(I'm still having periods, albeit irregular) and I've been off of it for six months and haven't had a night sweat since. I think when I checked, one of the side effects was excessive sweating. Also I started having very vivid nightmares which stopped once I was off it. As far as getting off of it, it was an absolute nightmare. It took me three months of very gradual withdrawal, and I experienced nausea ,dizziness, and brain zaps every time I went down in my dose. Also I experienced anger and impatience, which I am still dealing with. I read on the depression site that it took about a year after withdrawal for one girl before she felt herself again. There are people on there whose stories of withdrawal are even worse than mine. And if all that doesn't scare you, I gained 20 pounds. If I knew then what I know now, I never would have gone on Effexor.

● Progesterone cream will only make you feel better if it is counter-balancing a high level of estrogen. You will only feel better if your hormones are balanced. I also used progesterone cream for mild symptoms. After six months or so, I started having major symptoms and when I finally had my hormones tested (I had stopped using the progesterone cream by that time), all of my hormones were low. My guess is that part (not all) of my symptoms were exacerbated by the fact that I was using the cream, but was also low in other hormones, which made things even more off balance. You need to find a doctor who will test your hormones and, if you want to replace them, you can do so with bioidentical hormones, which you can have made specifically for you at a compounding pharmacy. You just need to find a doctor who does this sort of thing. Many more doctors are doing this now.

● I am taking DHEA (which I have read can have some effect on increasing estrogen and testosterone) and I was also using testosterone cream until just recently, along with a few other supplements. Regarding libido: Mine is much improved. For the first couple of weeks it was a little bit over the top, but it is calmed down and more normal. I stopped using the testosterone because it was making my hair fall out.

Q I have been in perimenopause since 1999. Two-and-a-half years ago I got hit with a bad case of anxiety. I started taking Buspar. It is a good anti-anxiety drug that is not addictive and has little side effects. Then this May the anxiety came back, right before a period. My doc upped the dose and I did well until the end of December. I had all the symptoms of bad PMS. anger, hostility, scalp breakouts, and anxiety. I hadn't had a period since the one in June, and I thought I was finally in menopause. But, no. Now I am on Celexa, an antidepressant. I just started it, so I don't know if it will help. I also go to the gym, take a good vitamin, flax seed oil (an omega 3), Promensil, and started using progesterone cream. Hopefully something will work.

Q I have been perimenopausal for two years and, although I have always been a bit anxious, I got really bad a year ago and had to have a lot of time off work. I don't like the thought of taking pills, so I decided to take up yoga and meditation. I do this at home, and I must say the difference in me has been amazing. Anxiety is all about relaxing your body, and although I still feel the anxiety now and again, it isn't nearly as bad.

Q I was on HRT for years (I am currently 55 and had first obvious symptoms of night sweats, etc., at age 39). A year ago I tried to wean myself off the pills by slowly reducing the dosage, but by the time I got to one-quarter of the original dosage, I was in flaming menopause again (brain fog, emotionally unstable, hot flashes, etc.). I told the doctor I was reconsidering my original decision and asked what we could do. He gave me a patch with Estradiol, which I think is bioidentical estrogen (I could be wrong). It gives a dosage of 25 micrograms per day (which cannot be compared to the dosage in a pill, as it enters the body by a different route). This is a relatively low dosage, which keeps the hot flashes to a minimum (not altogether gone, but tolerable), and allows my brain to function and my emotions to be more or less normal, that is, only as unstable as I was before I started going through menopause! As I cannot let any recipe alone, I've modified the usage to be: one patch lasts for six days instead of the prescribed three to four days, and I count three patches and then a six-day rest. I use the progesterone cream for the second and third patch weeks (that's six days patch only, 12 days patch and cream, and six days rest). So my cycle is 24 days, which is closer to what I had when I had normal periods. This lower dosage of estrogen is not enough for my vagina, so my doctor gave me some estrogen vaginal cream so I could have loving time with my hubby and not scream in pain and have vaginal and urinary infections afterward. I got tired of using the progesterone twice a day because it takes three to five minutes to rub the greasy stuff into my skin. So I figured that since I'm currently taking a low dosage of estrogen, I can get away with a low dosage of progesterone. I use it only in the mornings after I've washed up, and I eyeball what looks to me like a quarter teaspoon. My understanding is that the progesterone cream is not a substitute for estrogen. One of the books written by Dr Lee book covers restoring the balance when the body has too much estrogen and not enough progesterone. It may be that if your body has stopped producing estrogen entirely, the progesterone alone may help, but I don't know. I've lived long enough to be skeptical that any substance is a miracle cure for everybody. And go into overdrive when I read or hear that something has no side effects and can do only good things for everybody. Even diabetics who need insulin have to try different combinations of drugs and diet to see what works for them, and the life-saving insulin does have side effects that they have to take into consideration. I do feel better using the estrogen patch rather than the pills. I always felt like I was artificially medicated when I took the pills, especially during the progesterone part of the cycle. Depending on the formula, I often found my PMS symptoms coming on during that time, and I tried to alter the dosage to have a minimum amount of progesterone, just enough to counter the estrogen so I wouldn't get the heart attacks and other dire things which are threatened for folks who take estrogen alone. Now that I'm using the progesterone cream, I can tell that the hormones are affecting my body, but it's more subtle and I don't have PMS (well, you'll have to ask my hubby!) and I don't feel as though I'm artificially medicated. I'm not sure yet what to do in the long term. I assume I'll have to go off the hormones eventually, but I'm not ready yet.

I am 53 and my last period was in February 2006. I used to take progesterone cream, but I went off of it about a year ago. I feel better now than ever. I am off my antidepressant and all hormones. For some reason, my anxiety and weight got better when I got off of the cream, which I had used for over two years. Everyone is so individual. Also, since I came off it, I do not have that feeling like I am going to start my period any minute, like with bloating, cramps, and that feeling we all know so well. I am taking a blend of 5HTP, two tablets two hours before bedtime, and it seems to have helped my depression 99.9 percent now for months. I sleep well, too. The one thing I have noticed is my skin is starting to look aged, so I probably need estrogen of some type. I would consider going on something to help slow the aging process, but I have very few symptoms. I am telling you in hopes you will see light at the end of the tunnel. I believe it gets better as we get completely through it. I also follow an insulin-resistant diet and have lost 18 pounds. I feel really good on it. I notice when I eat sugar of any kind my heart pounds for about two hours and I am tired the next day. I also make myself walk every day, even if it is only for 15 to 20 minutes. I also use hand weights.

I just started on a prescription compounded hormone cream with testosterone included in it. I found that the dosage recommended to me made me nauseous and bloated. Instead of doing it twice a day, I went to once a day. That helped. I did find it helped my sex drive a little, though not a huge difference. I sort of feel that that the whole hormone thing is a pretty inexact science though because of the way our hormones fluctuate from day to day. I wasn't having hot flashes or night sweats and my periods are still pretty regular (at 54!), but I tested at zero for estrogen and testosterone when I had my hormones tested. So my gynecologist wanted me to try the cream. I think it's evened out my mood swings, and that alone has been worth it.

One month ago my doctor gave me a Depo Testotserone shot (monthly shot), and I couldn't wait for that stuff to wear off. It caused depression something terrible. I told my doctor that this was causing depression, and he said that DepoTestosterone doesn't cause depression. Well my next visit with him was last week and I took him what I had come across online about Depo Testosterone and its possible side effects. Sure as heck one of the side effects was depression. I showed him this and all he said was "I hate these online things." I told him I refuse to do another shot of that poison, so he prescribed me the bioidentical testosterone cream instead. I'm still debating about the testosterone cream, too. I mean will it also cause depression? I keep hearing good things about bioidentical hormone therapy, and I hear bad things about it as well. I mean, what happens when a person stops taking these bioidenticals? Do they have withdrawals from the stuff? I am sure if I ask my doctor he will give me the wrong answer as he did with the Depo Testosterone shot ordeal. Either way, I am still scared to try these two bioidentical creams, afraid it will bring back the depression.

After massive reading on the subject, here is what I've gleaned: Estrogen can be cancer causing, bioidentical or not. Many women are prescribed estrogen (like the pill) as a first route to controlling menopausal problems without a doctor first testing to see if they are high or low in both estrogen and progesterone. Compounded estrogen, which is used on the skin, is normally considered fine since it is not absorbed at high levels. Progesterone is not considered cancer-causing although overuse of it could be a factor in cancer since overuse could also cause an upsurge of estrogen levels beyond what is considered normal for a woman. Excess use of estrogen can also be a factor in strokes and heart attacks in women since it can cause blood clots. Progesterone will not cause blood clots and is considered safe for use for women with a history of high blood pressure, heart problems, or clotting issues. I also agree that the best route is to have your hormones tested by a doctor and then have your progesterone compounded at a pharmacy rather than buying anything over the shelf. I would also start any of these products at the lowest possible level since often women use it at a potency far beyond what they actually need to control their symptoms.

I went to my OB/GYN yesterday and discussed my continuing menopause symptoms. I was still having hot flashes after more than three years. She said some women continue to have them forever! We talked about HRT. She basically said it's an individual decision based on how serious your symptoms are, i.e., are they interrupting your life or are they just annoying. You have to weigh the benefits vs. the risks. Some women decide to take the risk; some just learn to deal with symptoms. She said to figure out what makes the hot flashes worse and avoid them (i.e., stress, wine, caffeine, etc.) and try to do more stuff that gets your mind off them (i.e., exercise, things you enjoy, etc.). After I get mamo and PAP results, she said if I really feel I need to go on HRT, she'll prescribe something. I think the most important thing she said is that different things work for different people. Some women benefit from progesterone cream, some don't, some can just take vitamins, some can use soy, you have to see what works for you. She recommended starting with the things with the least risk (i.e., soy, black cohosh, estroven, etc.). HRT should be the last resort.

I am 52 and ended birth control pills after taking them for nine months. They worked great to stop the heavy bleeding I was having. The other symptoms didn't change much. I still had headaches, heart palpitations, acne, anxiety, itchy skin, muscle aches, just to name a few. The pill wasn't the magic bullet I had hoped for, but it sure made my periods better. If heavy bleeding is one of your problems, I would consider the pill. Many women have good luck with it helping other symptoms, too, I guess I just wasn't one of the lucky ones.

About five years ago I quit breastfeeding my last child and with the return of my periods I began getting dizzy right before or during my period. I was 43 years old. It has been happening sporadically ever since. In the beginning, it happened every month for about six months. Then it didn't happen for several months. It has been like that. Sometimes an episode is very mild where it is very light and mostly unnoticeable and lasts only a few days. Sometimes they last ten days and are accompanied by extreme fatigue and I am bedridden for at least 24 hours, so dizzy that I have to put my head down on its side to feel somewhat balanced. For several other days I lay down whenever possible. The bad episodes are really bad. I went on the pill ten months ago to try to level out my hormones, but I just had one of my worst episodes while on the pill. I've read that it might be low blood sugar as well. This condition can be completely debilitating.

I am now dealing with the hormones. I will be 50 next month, but I have had irregular periods for about two years. PMS started long ago for me, so some symptoms are not unfamiliar. I have some hot flashes, though not really bad. I haven't had a period since June. I have been on bioidentical hormone cream for two years. I was diagnosed with low progesterone and a little high estrogen and low testosterone. But since my periods have stopped (for now), I bet my estrogen is way low, too. I did a saliva test for my first round of cream and recently did another to see where I am now. The test results will be in next week. I wanted to go this route because of a personal friend of mine. She had a hysterectomy at age 34 because of fibroid tumors, was put on HRT, and for several years endured headaches, fibrocystic lumps in her breasts and beginning stages of arthritis. She learned of the natural hormone creams and found a doctor who understands them and he slowly weaned her off of the HRT. Now she is actively involved in educating other women about the dangers of traditional HRT and the benefits of all natural bio-identical creams and the differences.

I was hit really hard by perimenopause symptoms last fall. I suddenly had light-headedness, nausea, heart palpitations, tingling/numbness in my fingers and toes, exhaustion beyond belief, body aches all over, massive weight loss due to the nausea, and my worst symptom, anxiety. The anxiety was so bad that I couldn't sleep at night. I kept believing that I had every illness known to mankind. I was convinced I was dying. One week it would be from ALS, the next heart disease, then cancer. It was horrible. I was going to the doctor every week for symptoms that had me believing that I was dying. My doctor put me on Clonanzapam for the anxiety, which did help, but I couldn't stand the dead, fogged-up feeling it left me with. It was all I could do to get through each day. I still had the body aches, tingling, and feelings of jumpiness inside. I went off the Clonanzapam and started taking Omega 3s, B stress supplements, and magnesium. I also began an exercise program. That all helped but still each month I would go through periods where the tingling and feelings of jumpiness and anxiety were unbearable. I felt like I was exploding inside. I decided to try Natural Progesterone Cream about three months ago, and I also started going to a chiropractor. I have to say that right now, for the first time in over a year, I feel normal. The anxiety is completely gone, my body doesn't ache all over anymore, and I have energy again. I feel like I did years ago. I don't know if it's the progesterone doing it and I'm not sure how long I want to stay on the cream since I worry that not enough testing has been done on it long term. I do like feeling normal though. I can't take anything with estrogen in it because I have a blood clotting problem. Apparently, progesterone is considered safe for people with blood clotting problems. I have no clue if it's the progesterone doing the trick, but I'm enjoying feeling like a normal person again.

● I use progesterone cream for anxiety, one quarter teaspoon twice a day of Emerita's Pro-Gest. I buy it at a health food store. I know everyone's system and hormone balances are different, but for me the progesterone cream works wonders. I lived with terrible anxiety, insomnia, and heart palpitations for over a year (along with a lot of other perimenopause symptoms) and I had no idea it was caused by perimenopause. Once I finally figured out I was in perimenopause, I decided to try progesterone cream, with the blessings of my gynecologist. Within two weeks of starting the cream, I was 95 percent anxiety and palpitation free. It's been two-and-a-half months now and, although I still have the occasional heart palpitations and hot flashes, their intensity is very much reduced and I am sleeping so much better and I am free of that awful anxiety.

● I took Yaz for three months for perimenopause symptoms. Initially, I felt a sense of relief. I had been suffering with perimenopause symptoms for over a year, and I was in pretty bad shape. The hardest things for me were the mood swings and anxiety that could turn into almost a rage. My relationships were suffering. I didn't want to take hormones, but I was desperate. Anyhow, like I said, initially I really did feel relief. However, it didn't turn out to be the cure-all I had hoped for. I really hate to tell you this, but I also noticed hair loss. Recently (a month ago) I added Lexapro, 10 mg., which has made a huge difference, so I stopped the Yaz about a week ago after the cycle was done. I go to the doctor in a couple of weeks, and I plan to tell her I'm just going to stick with Lexapro for now, unless a bunch of symptoms start bothering me. The hair loss on the Yaz really ticked me off, as I don't need to feel worse about my aging looks than I already do.

● I'm in the beginning stages of perimenopause, at 40 years old. It's been about a year, and I feared it would take its toll on my marriage. I finally agreed to start taking Lexapro, like

Mistyeyze I realized it's time to take the initiative to help myself feel better. I fought to avoid any medication but realized it could be a very long road to menopause and wasn't willing to risk my marriage by being so miserable. My husband did all he could to understand what was happening, but he became just as frustrated as I was because he couldn't find any way to help, he just sensed the mood and tip-toed around me. We started to avoid each other rather than risk having an argument or watching a teary outburst for no reason. I've been taking Lexapro for approximately four weeks, and it's changed my life! Now I feel silly that I tried to convince everyone I was strong enough to deal with all of this without it. I'm back to my old self, happy, ambitious, and it's been a huge relief. I was told that it's so gradual that you don't even realize how improved you've become until you look back on the hell you went through. I started to feel a difference approximately two weeks into it, as far as the hot flashes, sleep problems, etc., go. A few women I know along with my gynecologist strongly recommend Remifemin. My gynecologist told me that this brand is regulated by the FDA; if it says 20 mg. (for example), it is, unlike the others that may be only 17 mg. in one tab, 19 mg. in another. That also applies to the black cohosh found in the herbal section of pharmacy, GNC, etc. I added Remifemin to treatment and only had mild hot flashes the day or two prior to my period and getting a better night's sleep. Perimenopause and menopause can take over our emotional and physical state plus anyone involved watching us suffer.

On my doctor's recommendation, I went to a local pharmacy (which is also a compounding pharmacy) and picked up a saliva test kit. When I got the results back, the compounding pharmacy mixed a bioidentical solution based on my test results tailored just for me. It comes in a cream, is relatively inexpensive, and works wonderfully. It was well worth the effort and I'm sure it's much better for my body than the synthetic versions.

I tried the natural progestrone cream off and on for several years. I never have had any luck with it. When I started back on it this fall to try to help with ovarian cysts and heavy periods, it made things worse. I finally started on birth control pills to stop the bleeding. Some women swear by the cream, others like me hate it. I guess it's different for everybody. If you don't feel like your getting the results you want, stop it for a while. I have read where your body needs a break from the cream every six months.

Q I've had the Estring since last summer and can't be happier with it. I had weaned myself (with my doctor's approval) off hormone therapy, and the ring is a great solution for me for localized symptoms. I'm 55 and have been menopausal for about four years. I highly recommend it if you want estrogen only "where you need it," and not taken orally. It's absolutely a great product. I have been using the Vivelle Dot for about a year. It is a bioidentical hormone patch. I started on .75 and now cut it in half. I had been on the Climara patch, also a bioidentical, but didn't care for it because it was changed to one a week whereas the Vivelle Dot is changed to two times a week. I had a hard time keeping the Climara patch on the whole week. I have not had any problems (knock on wood) with the patch and have contemplated weaning myself off, but am afraid of spiraling downhill again! (I like knowing that I have the other half to add if I need to). The only drawback is the sticky residue it leaves on your hips. It is helpful to wipe the area first with an alcohol swab to get the best "stickiness." I have had a few hot flashes, but not like I had before. The anxiety has much improved, but I am also on 10 mgs. of Lexapro a day as well as fish oil three times a day. Oh, another thing, the Vivelle Dot I am on is estrogen only because I had a partially hysterectomy and was told I did not need the progesterone.

Q I have been using bioidentical hormones for about eight months. The first two to three months, my periods were so wacky I wasn't really getting the proper doses. So, we switched the methods so that I used the cream at a lower dose the first half of my cycle, then increased the dose the latter half (when hormone levels usually drop). It contains estrogen, progesterone, and testosterone, and I take DHEA orally. From that point, I noticed some changes within a month, like having more energy, less insomnia, fewer headaches, less anxiety. It probably took more like three to four months where I started feeling better overall with my heart not racing as much, etc. It's been up and down overall because my hormones fluctuate with my cycles. I had a second saliva test about two months ago, and my estrogen and testosterone were a little high, so I got a new prescription compounded, which I've been on this past week. I've noticed this past month, I seem to be experiencing a little more anxiety (like this morning my chest feels tight and I'm getting a little of the "fight or flight" feeling and there is no reason for it). So, I'm wondering if I have a little too much estrogen floating in my system. Hopefully, in the next week or so, things will get better. Of course, I'm also on the "downhill slide" to my period, which usually causes some or all symptoms to flare up.

🔊 I am on HRT. I am in menopause due to a hysterectomy ten months ago at the age of 39. I am now 40 years old. I am on a very low dose of Estroderm 0.05 mg. patch that I change twice a week. It does help, but there are still times I do suffer. My OB wants me to try it three times a week, but I am trying not to. Then again, spring is coming and it is getting more difficult for me. I am also on Xanax 0.25 mg. three times a day when needed. This helps for the anxiety and the heart palpitations. I started this problem about five months after my surgery. I was also told it could help for the hot flashes and night sweats.

🔊 I have sore scaly spots on my scalp. Actually I just noticed this morning a new one that almost feels like a bump. I've been to a dermatologist for this, and she says it folliculitis. I guess that's something like an ingrown hair follicle. Anyway, it really hurts at times. She said to use T-gel shampoo, but that really strips the color from my hair, so I found Jason's organic scalp balancing shampoo at the health food store. It costs less than the T-gel and is much gentler. I ran out, and now I'm having the issue again, so that figures. I don't know if it's menopause related, but I didn't seem to get this until I turned about 46, and I got adult acne as well. I'm 49 now and still get irregular periods.

🔊 I am 53 and at this point have not had my period for eight months, the longest I have gone without it. Three years ago I had the stomach issues and did not realize it was even part of perimenopause. Then a book called *The Pause* was recommended, and it goes through each symptom, why you have the symptom, and also how to deal with it. If you haven't read it,

I highly recommend it, as I found it helpful to get answers to why my hormones would be doing these things. From what I have read, we have estrogen receptors in the stomach that cause the problems. As for the hot flashes, I have had maybe one. So not everyone gets them. Unfortunately that is all we were told about. But our hormones affect us in so many other ways besides hot flashes. I don't know why the stomach issues subsided for me, but they did.

I have had the palpitations and still have the stomach problems. They go away for a while but always come back. My muscle pain moves around. It usually stays in one spot for about a month and then moves to another one. It is really crazy. I am four years without a period. The symptoms for me started after I didn't have a period for one year. Then the next two years were hell. I had some time off (about two years) when I felt good most of the time. Now, they are back. It is not fun.

I was 55 in September and will actually be two years without a period in January. The hot flashes have gone within the last six months, the PMS went at about the same time as the last period, so I am much more on an even keel, very few ups and downs. Sleep is still a bit of a problem, but I've given up worrying about that. I sleep when I'm tired now, maybe after two or three restless nights. The menopause supplements I used to use were discontinued, and I couldn't find any without the soya isoflavins, which I didn't ever take, so I decided about two or three months ago to see how I went on without any, and so far so good! I'm at the point of deciding what supplements I should now be taking to keep myself healthy, being post menopausal (you've no idea how good it is to write that!). I guess I should maybe take some calcium and omega 3, but I need to check up on all that. You do come through it, you do feel normal again. All you ladies who are in the middle of it, take heart, life does settle down and you will be fine, even better than fine, you will feel great that it's all over!

I started having headaches (migraines, actually) at the very beginning—I am still a newbie—about one year ago. I noticed a pattern where the migraines would occur anytime from three days prior until two or three days into my period. I asked my gynecologist, and he said they are hormonal headaches or migraines. He gave me a prescription for Imitrex. He said some women are prone to these headaches at times when hormones are out of whack, such as puberty, pregnancy, and menopause. I know when I feel one coming on. I usually start to get a little foggy, really sensitive to light and sound, and sometimes see flashes. Before I started the Imitrex, or when I've forgotten to refill, what would follow the warning signs would be horrible throbbing pain, like my head was going to explode, and usually nausea and a feeling of low-grade fever. I don't have to take the Imitrex every day. It's not a maintenance medication. I just take it as soon as I feel one coming, and it seems to pretty much stop it.

I have terrible water retention. I normally gain five to seven pounds of water when I'm PMSing. I take over-the-counter stuff for PMS symptoms, and it helps very little. My mom says that she also had terrible water retention when she was about to go through the change. Last month I waited an extra three weeks to start my period. I had PMS weight gain for three weeks instead of the normal five to seven days. I have even bought several items of clothing a size larger to wear on these days because my regular clothes won't fit. It's the most horrible symptom that I have. Cucumbers and asparagus help with water retention, but I have to eat it every day while retaining.

I am 49, and I started going through perimenopause around 43. I actually got fired from my job because I was having bad heavy periods, memory problems, and mood swings. Being fired only increased my already sleepless nights. I went the gamut of flooding, heavy periods, fibroids, hot flashes, weight gain, memory problems, crying over everything, and then last year, things started to change. My periods went from being heavy and plentiful to very sparse, I started skipping months, and now I seem to be over them altogether. I am sleeping really good now, have lost my fibroid belly, although I still have some flab I want to get rid of. But, I think the thing of us following our mother's is true. My mom went through menopause at 49, and now here I am. So, my advice, look into natural Progesterone cream, eat a healthy diet, and exercise, even if you don't feel like it now. It will pay off.

● I am a 51 year old and a very active female runner with my period stopping two months ago and hot flashes started immediately. I am currently taking Gabapentin and at 900 mg. They did not seem to help that much. I was still having seven or eight hot flashes a day and night sweats all the time. I am have now increased to 1,800 mg. and will see how that goes. I have read that you need 2,400 mg. to equal the effect of estrogen. I had breast cancer ten years ago with receptor positive and my doctor does not recommend any hormone treatments for fear of a recurrence.

● When I was 37, I started having periods every other week, lasting seven days, extremely heavy, and I would go through tampons every hour. I would do this for two or three months, then return to normal for two or three months. I went to the doctor and he did a biopsy, which was normal, and tested my hormones, which were normal. One year later, my periods suddenly stopped. I did not have any hot flashes or night sweats. My only symptom has been that I started having migraines. My hormones were tested and were all at post-menopause levels. My estrogen was undetectable. When menopause occurs before age 40, it is called Premature Ovarian Failure. And believe it or not, you can still get a period. The tests needed are a Day 3 Estradiol, FSH and LH. To confirm POF, you must test at menopausal levels two months. Ask for the test and don't let them tell you that you are too young. Since I was diagnosed, I have found a lot of women have this. I wouldn't be too worried about not having a period unless you want to conceive or are having symptoms. But you really should get tested to confirm any problems. Having a premature menopause can cause early bone loss. Make sure to get plenty of calcium. My doctor has me on 1,500 mg. a day plus Boniva once a month.

● I am nearly 52 and started the menopause at 47. So far I haven't noticed that I have withered or bloated, thank goodness. I am the same weight as I was before all this started and, although I have noticed a slight thickening around my waist, that's about it really. I don't take HRT or any supplements, but I do eat a good diet and do five miles a day on the treadmill, which has really helped a lot.

Q   I have just turned 52 and have been missing periods for the last two years. The first time was for three months and I, too, took an FSH test myself. It was also negative. I then had my periods for a few months and stopped again for about seven months. To my surprise they returned again and I had them for about four months. That was ten months ago, and I have been period free for ten months now. I did do another test in between, but it was still negative. I thought I would leave it until I had missed my periods for one year.

Q   I was referred to the endocrinologist by my primary care doctor because he just couldn't figure out why I was having so many weird symptoms and just didn't link it all to menopause. The endocrinologist really wasn't able to prescribe anything to help the symptoms (I refused HRT), but he certainly helped me to calm down about why I was feeling so bad. He was the one who explained to me that hormonal fluctuations in women can bring about a multitude of symptoms, that it seems to be different for everyone, and that the anxiety it creates can make it worse. So he helped me to understand what was happening with my body, and once I knew what it was (I didn't have a fatal disease!), I was able to just mentally handle it better. The endocrinologist did run a more in-depth battery of blood tests than my other doctor, which all came back normal, and verified that I was indeed entering menopause. If you think that seeing an endocrinologist will help give you peace of mind and rule out that anything else is wrong, then I say it is well worth it. It certainly helped me! Also, I was very fortunate to have been referred to this particular endocrinologist. He was patient, he listened to me, and he didn't dismiss me as being over emotional.

Q   I was suffering from stomach issues a year ago last October. I had the extreme nausea (I lost 22 pounds almost overnight), the burning sensation in my hands and feet, exhaustion beyond belief, tingling in my head, headaches, a shaky feeling inside, and anxiety. Truly, I thought I was dying. It lasted for about ten months, but I do have a great improvement now. I went on anti-anxiety medications for several months until I felt ready to cope with it all. I started using fish oils, B Stress complex and magnesium which did take the edge off it to some degree, although I was still bothered so badly by the burning sensation in my hands and feet and I still had terrible bouts with nausea. I can't do any form of estrogen since I have blood clotting issues, so I went with the natural progesterone cream instead. It took about two months before I saw results. I have scarcely any problems anymore. I get a minute bit of tingling in my feet around my period but nothing like it used to be. The nausea is completely gone, and I don't have any anxiety anymore. It feels so great to feel pretty normal.

About eight years ago, I started losing a lot of hair. As my hair was extremely thick, it was only noticeable to me. I started using Rogaine and have used it faithfully ever since. It did stop the hair loss. The first box will cost you $19.99, but every box has a $5 coupon in it, and I figured I was worth $14.99 a month. Fast forward to now. I skipped through perimenopause with only bitchiness and weight gain. I had no hot flashes, and because I had a partial hysterectomy in 1996, I had no periods. Still there are so many problems. I wish I had seen a doctor when the hair loss started. You really need to get your thyroid checked. I just started thyroid medicine. My hands and feet are just freezing. It isn't constant, but I will just suddenly get really cold, and even with two pair of socks on I cannot get warm. Also, I suggest you find a female doctor. In my experience, male doctors are not much interested in menopause problems. I have suffered for the last two years until I changed doctors.

I have to say that my anxiety was horrific last year. I couldn't sleep nights, I felt like I couldn't sit still. I was such a mess. I lost vast amounts of weight from the constant anxiety and was so exhausted that I could barely make it through the day. I'm not a candidate for the low dose pill or HRT since I'm prone to blood clots. I've come completely around the corner since then. I tried three different kinds of anxiety medications and can't say I loved any of them. The best was Klonopin, but it still left me exhausted. It did help me sleep though and was the first step to getting my life back together. It gave me the ability to manage the anxiety while I looked for other avenues that didn't require remaining on anxiety medications while I worked my way through six years of perimenopause. The best changes I made were to make sure that I regularly exercised, including both aerobic and weight work. I added a B stress vitamin, Omega

3's, flax seed oil, and magnesium to my regimen. I eliminated caffeine completely since it just threw my anxiety levels over the edge. I did start sleeping better and the worst edge was taken off my anxiety by doing all this. I made sure my diet was filled with fresh fruit, veggies, low fat protein and carbs that were low on the glycemic index. It's been mentioned that the anxiety is caused by low progesterone. I had read that as well, so I added in natural progesterone cream which was the final touch that fixed the remaining problems. I have absolutely no anxiety now, no tingling in my hands and feet, I've gotten back to normal weight levels and feel fantastic. I feel like my normal self again, full of energy and ready to go all day and night.

FSH levels differ depending on what day of the month they are tested on. The general base is to get a cycle day 3 FSH. Anything under a level 10 is considered to be within normal levels that would allow for pregnancy to occur. Anything over a level 10 means that the ovarian reserve is getting low or the remaining eggs are of poor quality. FSH levels can also differ from month to month. A woman trying to get pregnant could well get an FSH level of 15 one month and would have a poor chance of achieving pregnancy but could get a level of 9.5 the next month and achieve pregnancy. If you are testing for menopause, the most accurate results occur after you have ceased to have a period. A woman with an FSH of 40 for instance would be considered to have a very poor remaining ovarian reserve but could still get pregnant if she happened to ovulate one of her few remaining good eggs. Testing FSH levels to determine if you are perimenopausal is considered to be highly inaccurate since the levels can vary so much depending on egg quality and quantity. A result of 4.7 on cycle day 3 would be like hitting a gold mine for a woman trying to get pregnant. On the cycle that I got pregnant with my youngest son, my FSH levels were 7.5 on day 3.

I have been experiencing dry mouth for six months. People tell me to take small sips of water, but I find that doesn't work. The problem is getting my saliva back. I find chewing gum every hour helps. Sometimes I need to chew several times during the hour, depending on how dry my mouth is. (Orbit sugarfree spearmint is my favorite). Eventually I feel the moisture returning to my mouth. It starts from the rear sides and works it way forward and I am able to swallow again.

● I am 45 and have recently discovered I have been going through perimenopause for the past year after going to specialist after specialist with a variety of symptoms. I also have gastritis and GERD (reflux) and have taken Aciphex for years. I have had constipation a lot over the last year, and the last time I went for a colonoscopy, they found I had developed diverticulosis. My doctor told me that it is extremely important to keep the bowels flowing to avoid making things worse (diverticulitis—infection of bowels), that diverticulosis cannot be healed but can get worse, and that I need to be taking fiber supplements to avoid constipation. I take the generic brand of Metamucil capsules (five per day twice a day), and I am regular now. So far I haven't figured out a way to avoid the bloating though, which I see is a normal symptom of perimenopause.

● My daughter works for eye doctors and said vision changes are very common during perimenopause years due to changing hormones. Also your eyes will produce less natural tears, making it harder to wear contact lenses. You got pushed into all the changes with a hysterectomy and taking HRT. I would talk with your eye doctor and see if an exam would help. They might recommend waiting several months to see if your hormone levels stabilize a bit before doing an exam. My daughter is pregnant and having a terrible time with her contacts. Her doctors won't change the strength of her glasses or contacts until she delivers because of her changing hormones. The same thing happens to us in perimenopause, with changing hormones, but thank goodness we're not pregnant!

● Sometimes at perimenopause, women develop dry eyes (as well as other dryness issues increasing). If you haven't seen an eye doctor, I'd do that, just to see if there is a problem with tear production. In the meantime, some artificial tears might help. Try to stay away from ones in bottles, or with preservative, as contamination can occur with the bottles, and preservatives can irritate. Look for individual vials with no preservatives, if you try them. It may be perimenopause, or it can be allergy, or it can be caused by any medications you're taking. I tried HRT for one week and had this sore gritty feeling happen. A good ophthalmologist can identify any problems.

🗨 I am 51 as of yesterday. July will be two years since my last period. At the end of August or early September, I noticed that my tongue felt as if I had scalded it, like if you drink something really hot. It was terrible. Also, my lips were cracked at the corners. Some days I only had the burning tongue, others just cracked lips, then some days both. It was the tip of my tongue that really burned for me. I read up a lot and found that this could be a symptom of menopause, but it could be other things as well, such as burning mouth syndrome, Sjögren's Syndrome. I really think what was bothering me was BMS, not Sjögren's Syndrome. I started taking vitamin B complex vitamins and it is practically gone, or at least at a level I can live with. On a one to twn scale, at first it was a ten that being bad. Now I can say it is at a one. The only other thing that bothers my mouth now is I always have a weird taste in my mouth, bitter, or somewhat metallic. I have suffered with a lot of symptoms of menopause, such as hot flashes, night sweats, the list goes on.

🗨 Here is my list of symptoms, it is not continual, in that I am not having these symptoms all the time but the past few years have had them: night sweats (more so a few months ago, with palpitations when I first got them, but now I only get them occasionally and not badly; prolonged PMS (meaning everything I normally would get with PMS—mood swings, anxiety, feeling tired—again not as bad now but was really at a peak this March and early April); cramps are usual before my period but I can get them a bit week before ; periods used to be every 28 days but in my early to mid-forties (I just turned 50 this year), they got to be where I could get them 22 to 24 days apart, and two times last year it came at day 40 and then one cycle came on day 50 (this year it has been day 25 until two months ago when I got it at day 31; note that flow is very short for the most part, only three days, and I have had times where it will come for two days, then nothing and then reappear a few days later, just lightly or brownish discharge; breast tenderness (although this is normal for me with my period and it comes only at that time); intestinal discomfort, with diarrhea at times a week before my period (more of an irritable bowel and gas in perimenopause in general but it seems to be better now, thankfully); aching at the time of what would be ovulation, in the area of ovaries and also referred type of aching in that area and above; and a back problem that I have (unrelated to perimenopause) is at times more flared up during cycle. My only complaint until this early March was just the shorter times between cycles and a bit more PMS issues. Then March came and anxiety was rampant. My doctor gave me Xanax to take as needed. My intestines were very much in an uproar. I do think my anxiety really had a lot to do with this, as it creates acidity in our system when we stress. I did not feel like myself during all of March and into the beginning of April. Then later April to now has been much better. I don't know what to attribute that to. I am taking vitamin B complex every morning and Estroven vitamins (which the doctor recommended). I am able to get back into a routine of exercise, which I hadn't been able to do due to back and ankle problems (jazzercize, bike at gym, and pilates). I have been reading a lot about the symptoms of perimenopause, and this has helped ease my anxiety. In general my perimenopause has been mostly a prolonged feeling of PMS though.

I will be 49 in October. I have one son soon to be 17 and have been with my boyfriend 13 years. I am lucky to have been able to be a stay-at-home mom since he was born. I spend a lot of my time taking care of my mother and my family, and I spend too much time on the computer at night. I always had regular periods, every 28 days, and never missed but had the usual PMS with back and leg aches. That was until about three years ago when periods came 24-26 days apart and the cramps and PMS were worse. The last couple of years my symptoms got worse, and the last year has been miserable. Here is my list that I can think of:

- Periods closer and more intense; missed three in the last year. Cramps at any time and the feeling I am getting my period any time
- Tingling in hands when I am on a computer for a while;
- Tingling in feet like lack of circulation;
- Dry skin;
- Gray hairs caught up with me;
- Brown spots on face and arms;
- Crashing fatigue;

- Insomnia;
- Reflux feeling of something in my throat;
- Anxiety, nervousness, always worried about my health and my Mother's;
- Worry so much about my son that I am driving him crazy and away; I call him constantly when he is not home, wanting to know what he's doing;
- Excess gas;
- Weight gain;
- I started smoking again even though it makes me feel awful;
- Nausea sometimes in the morning, freak out I may be pregnant;
- Craving for chocolate chip cookies warm from the oven at 1:00 a.m.;
- Frequent headaches;
- Lack of energy and not wanting to do anything outside of the house;
- Sadness, not so much depression, and very emotional; I cry over a Kleenex commercial;
- No sexual desire the last year or so, it's almost repulsive;
- The one that is currently freaking me out is my hips, thighs, and legs ache so bad the last few months mostly all the time, and sometimes when I walk even short distance they hurt and I feel like I am ninety;
- And let me not forget, forgetful and spacey.

The only thing I have not had is night sweats and hot flashes, but I think I had them in my late thirties. Also, my gums have gotten worse in the last six months. I am now rinsing every day with Listerine. When I sweat, I have an odor I never had before. For the last three months I have been taking multi super B max, magnesium, potassium, calcium/D, vitamin E, vitamin C, and fish oil concentrate. I don't know if all this really helps or not, but I know it does not cure and my skin is not as dry.

I'm 52 and it's been ten years since I went through it all. But still I have some symptoms. Right now they are:

- Insomnia (why I am on the computer so late at night until early morning);

- Don't sleep as much when I do (work at home);
- Dry skin, especially on the hands and feet;
- Itchy skin, such as hands and feet;
- Crawly skin sometimes, which I hate too;
- Skin thinning, which lack of estrogen causes, and lowering of Growth Hormone—HGH supplements and exercise have brought some of this back;
- Morning aches and pains;
- Heat and cold temps affect me more now than they used to, although I have warm hands;
- Loss of sex drive, as it's too dry down there and the walls are thinner for one reason and it hurts if my husband is too eager and foreplay is not long enough, although he is caring;
- Irritable at times;
- Some foods not agreeing with me anymore;
- Flatulence, yep; and
- Anxiety, in the beginning.

I am 49 years old. I have had my periods more frequently, now about every three weeks, although some months closer. They have been a lot heavier. The past week, though, I have been experiencing bad anxiety when I feel as though I can jump out of my skin. After reading a lot about this, I assume it has to do with my age and making my way to that wonderful thing all women get to experience—menopause. My sexual drive has been way down for a while now. That part really sucks. I have the breast pain from time to time also. I know you can be put on medication for this sort of thing, but I'm planning on riding it out as long as I can without the help of medication. I have learned that medications may take away one symptom but they can cause so many other side effects, so for me I really want to do this naturally. Hopefully I'll be like my mother and she didn't do that bad with menopause. The doctor keeps telling me I'll follow my mother pretty much the same, so we shall see.

This is day six without any hormones. I stopped my birth control pills and Vivelle in order to find out my FSH level and then decide what to do next. Tomorrow I have the blood work done and then I should know something in a couple of days. As far as symptoms go, I'm sitting here with the jitters, which I haven't had in almost a year, and I'm nervous, anxious, spacey, lightheaded, and tired. Although I have these symptoms, they are way better than what I've experienced in the last three years. Just knowing that all of this is hormone related and nothing terminal helps me to endure. Even though these symptoms are annoying realizing that they aren't as intense reassures me that the end is near. Once upon a time I couldn't go two days without taking my birth control pills, now I'm on day six! By the way, I've been taking flaxseed, primrose oil, soy isoflavone, lecithin, B6, calcium, and magnesium the last couple of days and they seem to help take the edge off many of my symptoms. They don't totally eliminate them, but I'm able to endure.

I think I've been in menopause forever. I am 60 and it isn't over yet. I think everyone has covered everything I've had, or am still having. The one thing that I've found to be the most helpful is magnesium. It helps with internal shaking, it stops mind racing, it helps with the feelings of coldness, it helps with vertigo and feeling like your ear is submerged in water or stuffed up, it helps calm your nerves, and takes away the jittery feelings, it helps with heart palpitations, it lessens the pain around your period. It helps with those times when you're depressed and gloomy and feel impending doom, bad dreams. They usually advise 500 magnesium and 1,000 to 1,200 calcium for menopausal women, but studies are showing that it should be more like a 1,000/1,000 mg. magnesium and calcium. The loss of estrogen seems to keep our bodies from picking up the magnesium and calcium in our system, and as time goes along we need more and more to compensate for the continual loss of estrogen. Also you should take vitamin D 400 mg. to help your body absorb the minerals better. A lot of doctors just don't have the nutritional background and so don't pay much attention to these symptoms unless it's a last resort, then again others are more informed. But even the tests they do use don't always show just how low you are. I was hospitalized before they actually found that I was low in magnesium. Magnesium will cause diarrhea if too much is taken, but it won't hurt you unless you decided to OD on the stuff.

I take spinning classes regularly and consistently, as well as weight train; and I take all antioxidants I can get my hands on plus the important-for-my age vitamins and minerals (such as calcium). I eat soy products (edamame, steamed young soy beans in pod) at least three times a week for the estrogen, although it is my understanding if breast cancer runs in the family, all estrogen high foods are out, fish (love all types of fish, plus sushi), veggies and chicken, and I drink lots of green tea (and chamomile when I feel I need or want to relax) as well as lots of water and no soda or diet products/drinks. Red wine is actually good, in moderation.

I have been using Stevia (natural sweetener used by diabetics which has no calories and does not affect blood sugar levels) for about four years, and I try to adhere to a healthy lifestyle (stress management for one). I don't take any prescription medications, my blood pressure is quite normal, cholesterol is total 180 with very low tryglicerides, and my weight is ideal for my height; although, without a doubt, I do have to work out harder than I used to in my late thirties or early forties to keep trim. My knees are not what they used to be, and I occasionally experience hip (left side, iliac crest) and lower back pain, so I have become more aware of my posture, but I view this, at least for now, as normal wear and tear. However, I find myself craving sweets more than ever before, so I reward myself occasionally (and moderately) with any of the following: 1) lowfat frozen yogurt or sorbet (there are many delicious flavors and types to choose from), 2) vanilla (my favorite) low fat ice cream, 3) a few small sized peppermint patties, 4) organic dark (not milk) chocolate. Another good habit I have adopted recently is taking wheatgrass shots (a drink). We can considerably lessen our discomforts by adhering to a healthy lifestyle and doing all we can nutritionally and by staying active, and most importantly, keeping a fresh outlook and positive attitude.

References

1. Walker ML (1995). "Menopause in female rhesus monkeys". *Am J Primatol* **35**: 59–71. doi:10.1002/ajp.1350350106.
2. McAuliffe K, Whitehead H (2005). "Eusociality, menopause and information in matrilineal whales". *Trends Ecol Evolution* **20**: 650. doi:10.1016/j.tree.2005.09.003.
3. David Reznick1, Michael Bryant, Donna Holmes. University of California Riverside, United States. david.reznick@ucr.edu
4. Bellipanni G, DI Marzo F, Blasi F, et al. Effects of melatonin in perimenopausal and menopausal women: our personal experience. 2005. Ann N Y Acad Sci 1057:393-402. DOI: 10.1196/annals.1356.030 **PMID 16399909**
5. Twiss JJ, Wegner J, Hunter M, Kelsay M, Rathe-Hart M, Salado W (2007). "Perimenopausal symptoms, quality of life, and health behaviors in users and nonusers of hormone therapy". *J Am Acad Nurse Pract* **19** (11): 602–13. doi:10.1111/j.1745-7599.2007.00260.x. PMID 17970860.
6. Freeman EW, Sammel MD, Lin H, *et al* (2007). "Symptoms associated with menopausal transition and reproductive hormones in midlife women". *Obstetrics and gynecology* **110** (2 Pt 1): 230–40. doi:10.1097/01.AOG.0000270153.59102.40 (inactive 2008-06-25). PMID 17666595.
7. Somjen D, Katzburg S, Knoll E, *et al* (May 2007). "DT56a (Femarelle): a natural selective estrogen receptor modulator (SERM)". *J. Steroid Biochem. Mol. Biol.* **104** (3-5): 252–8. doi:10.1016/j.jsbmb.2007.03.004. PMID 17428655.
8. http://en.wikipedia.org/wiki/Hormone_replacement_therapy_(menopause)#Types_of_Hormone_Replacement_Therapy Types
9. Menon U, Burnell M, Sharma A, *et al* (2007). "Decline in use of hormone therapy among postmenopausal women in the United Kingdom". *Menopause* **14** (3 Pt 1): 462–7. doi:10.1097/01.gme.0000243569.70946.9d. PMID 17237735.
10. Du Y, Dören M, Melchert HU, Scheidt-Nave C, Knopf H (2007). "Differences in menopausal hormone therapy use among women in Germany between 1998 and 2003". *BMC Womens Health* **7**: 19. doi:10.1186/1472-6874-7-19. PMID 17945013.
11. Watson J, Wise L, Green J (September 2007). "Prescribing of hormone therapy for menopause, tibolone, and bisphosphonates in women in the UK between 1991 and 2005". *Eur. J. Clin. Pharmacol.* **63** (9): 843–9. doi:10.1007/s00228-007-0320-6. PMID 17598097.
12. Clarke CA, Glaser SL, Uratsu CS, Selby JV, Kushi LH, Herrinton LJ (November 2006). "Recent declines in hormone therapy utilization and breast cancer incidence: clinical and

population-based evidence". *J. Clin. Oncol.* **24** (33): e49–50. doi:10.1200/JCO.2006.08.6504. PMID 17114650.

13. Ravdin PM, Cronin KA, Howlader N, *et al* (April 2007). "The decrease in breast-cancer incidence in 2003 in the United States". *N. Engl. J. Med.* **356** (16): 1670–4. doi:10.1056/NEJMsr070105. PMID 17442911.

14. Glass AG, Lacey JV, Carreon JD, Hoover RN (August 2007). "Breast cancer incidence, 1980-2006: combined roles of menopausal hormone therapy, screening mammography, and estrogen receptor status". *J. Natl. Cancer Inst.* **99** (15): 1152–61. doi:10.1093/jnci/djm059. PMID 17652280.

15. Smith NL, Heckbert SR, Lemaitre RN, *et al* (2004). "Esterified estrogens and conjugated equine estrogens and the risk of venous thrombosis". *JAMA* **292** (13): 1581–7. doi:10.1001/jama.292.13.1581. PMID 15467060.

16. "Bioidentical Hormones Come Of Age", Marcelle Pick, OB/GYN Nurse Practitioner; published March 24, 2004; updated June 7, 2007; retrieved June 13, 2007.

17. Jr, Guttuso T.; Kurlan, R.; McDermott, M. P.; Kieburtz, K. (2003), "Gabapentin's effects on hot flashes in postmenopausal women: a randomized controlled trial", *Obstetrics & Gynecology* **101**(2): 337–45, doi:10.1016/S0029-7844(02)02712-6, PMID 12576259

18. Yoles I, Yogev Y, Frenkel Y, Hirsch M, Nahum R, Kaplan B (2004). "Efficacy and safety of standard versus low-dose Femarelle (DT56a) for the treatment of menopausal symptoms". *Clin Exp Obstet Gynecol* **31** (2): 123–6. PMID 15266766.

19. Somjen D, Katzburg S, Knoll E, *et al* (May 2007). "DT56a (Femarelle): a natural selective estrogen receptor modulator (SERM)". *J. Steroid Biochem. Mol. Biol.* **104** (3-5): 252–8. doi:10.1016/j.jsbmb.2007.03.004. PMID 17428655.

20. Yoles I, Yogev Y, Frenkel Y, Nahum R, Hirsch M, Kaplan B (2003). "Tofupill/Femarelle (DT56a): a new phyto-selective estrogen receptor modulator-like substance for the treatment of postmenopausal bone loss". *Menopause* **10** (6): 522–5. doi:10.1097/01.GME.0000064864.58809.77. PMID 14627860.

21. Yoles I, Lilling G (January 2007). "Pharmacological doses of the natural phyto-SERM DT56a (Femarelle) have no effect on MCF-7 human breast cancer cell-line". *Eur. J. Obstet. Gynecol. Reprod. Biol.* **130** (1): 140–1. doi:10.1016/j.ejogrb.2006.02.010. PMID 16580119.

22. Somjen D, Yoles I (July 2003). "DT56a (Tofupill/Femarelle) selectively stimulates creatine kinase specific activity in skeletal tissues of rats but not in the uterus". *J. Steroid Biochem. Mol. Biol.* **86** (1): 93–8. PMID 12943748.

23. Oropeza MV, Orozco S, Ponce H, Campos MG (2005). "Tofupill lacks peripheral estrogen-like actions in the rat reproductive

tract". *Reprod. Toxicol.* **20** (2): 261–6. doi:10.1016/j.reprotox.2005.02.007. PMID 15878261.
24. Nir Y, Huang MI, Schnyer R, Chen B, Manber R. Stanford University School of Medicine, United States. amiryael@gmail.com
25. Cohen SM, Rousseau ME, Carey BL. University of Pittsburgh, 440 Victoria Bldg, 3500 Victoria St, Pittsburgh, PA 15261, USA. cohensu@pitt.edu
26. Zaborowska E, Brynhildsen J, Damberg S, Fredriksson M, Lindh-Astrand L, Nedstrand E, Wyon Y, Hammar M. Division of Obstetrics and Gynecology, Department of Molecular and Clinical Medicine, Faculty of Health Sciences, University Hospital, Linköping, Sweden.
27. Vincent A, Barton DL, Mandrekar JN, Cha SS, Zais T, Wahner-Roedler DL, Keppler MA, Kreitzer MJ, Loprinzi C. Mayo Clinic College of Medicine, Rochester, MN 55905, USA.
28. Fournier LR, Ryan Borchers TA, Robison LM, Wiediger M, Park JS, Chew BP, McGuire MK, Sclar DA, Skaer TL, Beerman KA. Department of Psychology, Washington State University, Pullman, WA 99164-4820, USA. Fournier@wsunix.wsu.edu
29. Sexual Lubrication from Discovery health

GNU Free Documentation License

0. PREAMBLE

The purpose of this License is to make a manual, textbook, or other functional and useful document "free" in the sense of freedom: to assure everyone the effective freedom to copy and redistribute it, with or without modifying it, either commercially or noncommercially. Secondarily, this License preserves for the author and publisher a way to get credit for their work, while not being considered responsible for modifications made by others.

This License is a kind of "copyleft", which means that derivative works of the document must themselves be free in the same sense. It complements the GNU General Public License, which is a copyleft license designed for free software.

We have designed this License in order to use it for manuals for free software, because free software needs free documentation: a free program should come with manuals providing the same freedoms that the software does. But this License is not limited to software manuals; it can be used for any textual work, regardless of subject matter or whether it is published as a printed book. We recommend this License principally for works whose purpose is instruction or reference.

1. APPLICABILITY AND DEFINITIONS

This License applies to any manual or other work, in any medium, that contains a notice placed by the copyright holder saying it can be distributed under the terms of this License. Such a notice grants a world-wide, royalty-free license, unlimited in duration, to use that work under the conditions stated herein. The "Document", herein, refers to any such manual or work. Any member of the public is a licensee, and is addressed as "you". You accept the license if you copy, modify or distribute the work in a way requiring permission under copyright law.

A "Modified Version" of the Document means any work containing the Document or a portion of it, either copied verbatim, or with modifications and/or translated into another language.

A "Secondary Section" is a named appendix or a front-matter section of the Document that deals exclusively with the relationship of the publishers or authors of the Document to the Document's overall subject (or to related matters) and contains nothing that could fall directly within that overall subject. (Thus, if the Document is in part a textbook of mathematics, a Secondary Section may not explain any mathematics.) The relationship could be a matter of historical connection with the subject or with related matters, or of legal, commercial, philosophical, ethical or political position regarding them.

The "Invariant Sections" are certain Secondary Sections whose titles are designated, as being those of Invariant Sections, in the notice that says that the Document is released under this License. If a section does not fit the above definition of Secondary then it is not allowed to be designated as Invariant. The Document may contain zero Invariant Sections. If the Document does not identify any Invariant Sections then there are none.

The "Cover Texts" are certain short passages of text that are listed, as Front-Cover Texts or Back-Cover Texts, in the notice that says that the Document is released under this License. A Front-Cover Text may be at most 5 words, and a Back-Cover Text may be at most 25 words.

A "Transparent" copy of the Document means a machine-readable copy, represented in a format whose specification is available to the general public, that is suitable for revising the document straightforwardly with generic text editors or (for images composed of pixels) generic paint programs or (for drawings) some widely available drawing editor, and that is suitable for input to text formatters or for automatic translation to a variety of formats suitable for input to text formatters. A copy made in an otherwise Transparent file format whose markup, or absence of markup, has been arranged to thwart or discourage subsequent modification by readers is not Transparent. An image format is not Transparent if used for any substantial amount of text. A copy that is not "Transparent" is called "Opaque".

Examples of suitable formats for Transparent copies include plain ASCII without markup, Texinfo input format, LaTeX input format, SGML or XML using a publicly available DTD, and standard-conforming simple HTML, PostScript or PDF designed for human modification. Examples of transparent image formats include PNG, XCF and JPG. Opaque formats include proprietary formats that can be read and edited only by proprietary word processors, SGML or XML for which the DTD and/or processing tools are not generally available, and the machine-generated HTML, PostScript or PDF produced by some word processors for output purposes only.

The "Title Page" means, for a printed book, the title page itself, plus such following pages as are needed to hold, legibly, the material this License requires to appear in the title page. For works in formats which do not have any title page as such, "Title Page" means the text near the most prominent appearance of the work's title, preceding the beginning of the body of the text.

A section "Entitled XYZ" means a named subunit of the Document whose title either is precisely XYZ or contains XYZ in parentheses following text that translates XYZ in another language. (Here XYZ stands for a specific section name mentioned below, such as "Acknowledgements", "Dedications", "Endorsements", or "History".) To "Preserve the Title" of such a section when you modify the Document means that it remains a section "Entitled XYZ" according to this definition.

The Document may include Warranty Disclaimers next to the notice which states that this License applies to the Document. These Warranty Disclaimers are considered to be included by reference in this License, but only as regards disclaiming warranties: any other implication that these Warranty Disclaimers may have is void and has no effect on the meaning of this License.

2. VERBATIM COPYING

You may copy and distribute the Document in any medium, either commercially or noncommercially, provided that this License, the copyright notices, and the license notice saying this License applies to the Document are reproduced in all copies, and that you add no other conditions whatsoever to those of this License. You may not use technical measures to obstruct or control the reading or further copying of the copies you make or distribute. However, you may accept compensation in exchange for copies. If you distribute a large enough number of copies you must also follow the conditions in section 3.

You may also lend copies, under the same conditions stated above, and you may publicly display copies.

3. COPYING IN QUANTITY

If you publish printed copies (or copies in media that commonly have printed covers) of the Document, numbering more than 100, and the Document's license notice requires Cover Texts, you must enclose the copies in covers that carry, clearly and legibly, all these Cover Texts: Front-Cover Texts on the front cover, and Back-Cover Texts on the back cover. Both covers must also clearly and legibly identify you as the publisher of these copies. The front cover must present the full title with all words of the title equally prominent and visible. You may add other material on the covers in addition. Copying with changes limited to the covers, as long as they preserve the title of the Document and satisfy these conditions, can be treated as verbatim copying in other respects.

If the required texts for either cover are too voluminous to fit legibly, you should put the first ones listed (as many as fit reasonably) on the actual cover, and continue the rest onto adjacent pages.

If you publish or distribute Opaque copies of the Document numbering more than 100, you must either include a machine-readable Transparent copy along with each Opaque copy, or state in or with each Opaque copy a computer-network location from which the general network-using public has access to download using public-standard network protocols a complete Transparent copy of the Document, free of added material. If you use the latter option, you must take reasonably prudent steps, when you begin distribution of Opaque copies in quantity, to ensure that this Transparent copy will remain thus accessible at the stated location until at least one year after the last time you distribute an Opaque copy (directly or through your agents or retailers) of that edition to the public.

It is requested, but not required, that you contact the authors of the Document well before redistributing any large number of copies, to give them a chance to provide you with an updated version of the Document.

4. MODIFICATIONS

You may copy and distribute a Modified Version of the Document under the conditions of sections 2 and 3 above, provided that you release the Modified Version under precisely this License, with the Modified Version filling the role of the Document, thus licensing distribution and modification of the Modified Version to whoever possesses a copy of it. In addition, you must do these things in the Modified Version:

A. Use in the Title Page (and on the covers, if any) a title distinct from that of the Document, and from those of previous versions (which should, if there were any, be listed in the History section of the Document). You may use the same title as a previous version if the original publisher of that version gives permission.

B. List on the Title Page, as authors, one or more persons or entities responsible for authorship of the modifications in the Modified Version, together with at least five of the principal authors of the Document (all of its principal authors, if it has fewer than five), unless they release you from this requirement.

C. State on the Title page the name of the publisher of the Modified Version, as the publisher.

D. Preserve all the copyright notices of the Document.

E. Add an appropriate copyright notice for your modifications adjacent to the other copyright notices.

F. Include, immediately after the copyright notices, a license notice giving the public permission to use the Modified Version under the terms of this License, in the form shown in the Addendum below.

G. Preserve in that license notice the full lists of Invariant Sections and required Cover Texts given in the Document's license notice.

H. Include an unaltered copy of this License.

I. Preserve the section Entitled "History", Preserve its Title, and add to it an item stating at least the title, year, new authors, and publisher of the Modified Version as given on the Title Page. If there is no section Entitled "History" in the Document, create one stating the title, year, authors, and publisher of the Document as given on its Title Page, then add an item describing the Modified Version as stated in the previous sentence.

J. Preserve the network location, if any, given in the Document for public access to a Transparent copy of the Document, and likewise the network locations given in the Document for previous versions it was based on. These may be placed in the "History" section. You may omit a network location for a work that was published at least four years before the Document itself, or if the original publisher of the version it refers to gives permission.

K. For any section entitled "Acknowledgements" or "Dedications", Preserve the Title of the section, and preserve in the section all the substance and tone of each of the contributor acknowledgements and/or dedications given therein.

L. Preserve all the Invariant Sections of the Document, unaltered in their text and in their titles. Section numbers or the equivalent are not considered part of the section titles.

M. Delete any section entitled "Endorsements". Such a section may not be included in the Modified Version.

N. Do not retitle any existing section to be entitled "Endorsements" or to conflict in title with any Invariant Section.

O. Preserve any Warranty Disclaimers.

If the Modified Version includes new front-matter sections or appendices that qualify as Secondary Sections and contain no material copied from the Document, you may at your option designate some or all of these sections as Invariant. To do this, add their titles to the list of Invariant Sections in the Modified Version's license notice. These titles must be distinct from any other section titles.

You may add a section entitled "Endorsements", provided it contains nothing but endorsements of your Modified Version by various parties-- for example, statements of peer review or that the text has been approved by an organization as the authoritative definition of a standard.

You may add a passage of up to five words as a Front-Cover Text, and a passage of up to 25 words as a Back-Cover Text, to the end of the list of Cover Texts in the Modified Version. Only one passage of Front-Cover Text and one of Back-Cover Text may be added by (or through arrangements made by) any one entity. If the Document already includes a Cover Text for the same cover, previously added by you or by arrangement made by the same entity you are acting on behalf of, you may not add another; but you may replace the old one, on explicit permission from the previous publisher that added the old one.

The author(s) and publisher(s) of the Document do not by this License give permission to use their names for publicity for or to assert or imply endorsement of any Modified Version.

5. COMBINING DOCUMENTS

You may combine the Document with other documents released under this License, under the terms defined in section 4 above for modified versions, provided that you include in the combination all of the Invariant Sections of all of the original documents, unmodified, and list them all as Invariant Sections of your combined work in its license notice, and that you preserve all their Warranty Disclaimers.

The combined work need only contain one copy of this License, and multiple identical Invariant Sections may be replaced with a single copy. If there are multiple Invariant Sections with the same name but different contents, make the title of each such section unique by adding at the end of it, in parentheses, the name of the original author or publisher of that section if known, or else a unique number. Make the same adjustment to the section titles in the list of Invariant Sections in the license notice of the combined work.

In the combination, you must combine any sections entitled "History" in the various original documents, forming one section entitled "History"; likewise combine any sections entitled "Acknowledgements", and any sections entitled "Dedications". You must delete all sections entitled "Endorsements."

6. COLLECTIONS OF DOCUMENTS

You may make a collection consisting of the Document and other documents released under this License, and replace the individual copies of this License in the various documents with a single copy that is included in the collection, provided that you follow the rules of this License for verbatim copying of each of the documents in all other respects.

You may extract a single document from such a collection, and distribute it individually under this License, provided you insert a copy of this License into the extracted document, and follow this License in all other respects regarding verbatim copying of that document.

7. AGGREGATION WITH INDEPENDENT WORKS

A compilation of the Document or its derivatives with other separate and independent documents or works, in or on a volume of a storage or distribution medium, is called an "aggregate" if the copyright resulting from the compilation is not used to limit the legal rights of the compilation's users beyond what the individual works permit. When the Document is included in an aggregate, this License does not apply to the other works in the aggregate which are not themselves derivative works of the Document.

If the Cover Text requirement of section 3 is applicable to these copies of the Document, then if the Document is less than one half of the entire aggregate, the Document's Cover Texts may be placed on covers that bracket the Document within the aggregate, or the electronic equivalent of covers if the Document is in electronic form. Otherwise they must appear on printed covers that bracket the whole aggregate.

8. TRANSLATION

Translation is considered a kind of modification, so you may distribute translations of the Document under the terms of section 4. Replacing Invariant Sections with translations requires special permission from their copyright holders, but you may include translations of some or all Invariant Sections in addition to the original versions of these Invariant Sections. You may include a translation of this License, and all the license notices in the Document, and any Warranty Disclaimers, provided that you also include the original English version of this License and the original versions of those notices and disclaimers. In case of a disagreement between the translation and the original version of this License or a notice or disclaimer, the original version will prevail.

If a section in the Document is entitled "Acknowledgements", "Dedications", or "History", the requirement (section 4) to Preserve its Title (section 1) will typically require changing the actual title.

9. TERMINATION

You may not copy, modify, sublicense, or distribute the Document except as expressly provided for under this License. Any other attempt to copy, modify, sublicense or distribute the Document is void, and will automatically terminate your rights under this License. However, parties who have received copies, or rights, from you under this License will not have their licenses terminated so long as such parties remain in full compliance.

10. FUTURE REVISIONS OF THIS LICENSE

The Free Software Foundation may publish new, revised versions of the GNU Free Documentation License from time to time. Such new versions will be similar in spirit to the present version, but may differ in detail to address new problems or concerns. See http://www.gnu.org/copyleft/.

Each version of the License is given a distinguishing version number. If the Document specifies that a particular numbered version of this License "or any later version" applies to it, you have the option of following the terms and conditions either of that specified version or of any later version that has been published (not as a draft) by the Free Software Foundation. If the Document does not specify a version number of this License, you may choose any version ever published (not as a draft) by the Free Software Foundation.